Are You A Moldy Patient?

Do you suffer from Thrush (yeasts)? Are you unwell in damp, musty environments? Are you intolerant of alcohol? Chemically sensitive? Sugar cravings? You could be a moldy patient, a term I invented for someone allergically sensitized and overrun by this family of organisms

Here's 35 years experience by one of the world's pioneer MDs in this field. Lots of self-help advice and places to turn.

You don't have to go on suffering. There is a path to health.

By

Keith Scott-Mumby MD, MB ChB, HMD, PhD

COPYRIGHT NOTICE

Published by:
Scott-Mumby Wellness Publishing
PO Box 371225, Las Vegas, NV 89137

10 9 8 7 6 5 4 3 2 1

Copyright © Dr Keith Scott-Mumby 2012
Dr Keith Scott-Mumby asserts the moral right to be identified as the author of this work.

ISBN 978-0-9884196-3-6

Keith Scott-Mumby MD, MB ChB, HMD, PhD

BEYOND CANDIDA

BREAKTHROUGH SOLUTIONS FOR CANDIDA, YEASTS, DYSBIOSIS AND MORE

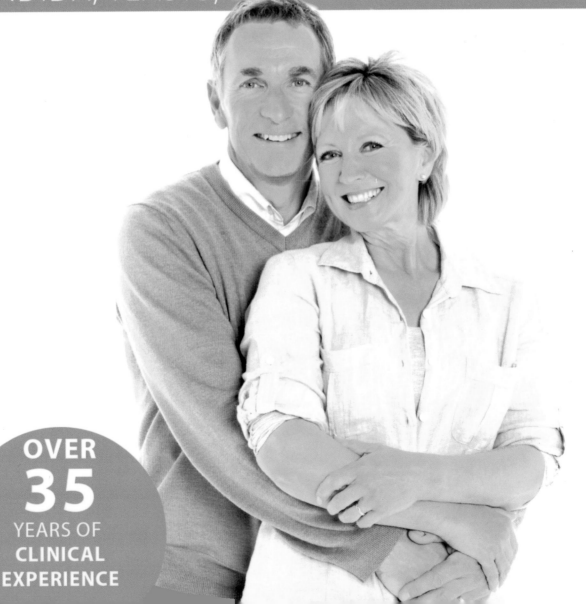

OVER 35 YEARS OF CLINICAL EXPERIENCE

Disclaimer

All content within this book is commentary or opinion and is protected under Free Speech laws in all the civilized world. The information herein is provided for educational and entertainment purposes only. It is not intended as a substitute for professional advice of any kind. Dr. Keith Scott-Mumby MD, PhD assumes no responsibility for the use or misuse of this material.

Keith Scott-Mumby intends that the information given should be accurate, however errors can occur. Therefore no warranty of any kind, whether expressed or implied, is given in relation to this information or any of the external services referred to.

In no event shall Professor Scott-Mumby be liable for any consequential damages arising out of any use of, or reliance on any content or materials contained herein, neither shall Professor Scott-Mumby be liable for any content of any external internet sites listed and services listed.

Always consult your own licensed medical practitioner if you are in any way concerned about your health. You must satisfy yourself of the validity of the professional qualifications of any health care provider you contact as a result of this book.

If you cannot agree to these terms, destroy the book if you downloaded it free, or ask for a refund and then destroy it if payment was made.

These are serious issues and intense pressure often falls on publishers of such needed information, from parties who do not wish you to know anything other than what they tell you is true. We ask you not to create problems by irresponsible use or spread of this valuable information.

All trademarks, registered trademarks and service marks mentioned in the book are the property of their respective owners.

Contents

Introduction

If you are suffering from a yeast infection, aka. Candida or Candidiasis, then this book is going to alleviate your fears and give you the practical answers to your problems. It doesn't matter if you have a mild infection or a very severe case, the information inside this book will help you.

You will learn it's part of a bigger problem: mold sensitivity. People with this condition tend to get thrush, athlete's foot, jock itch and those lousy disfiguring toenails you hate so much. Often it goes along with food allergies, chemical intolerance and mercury overload.

I've had over 35 years experience as a physician, treating this very difficult condition and the information contained in this book is going to allow you to completely get on top of the yeast infection that you currently have. Maybe you will start to make progress for the first time.

There is a LOT of information here and you need to get educated. This is the most complete book of its kind on the market. Knowledge will help you bring it around and come out right.

It's also important to know that you are not alone. It is very common for people of all backgrounds and ages to develop yeast infection at some point during their lifetime. Of course, the condition is very irritable and annoying, and you want to expel it as soon as possible.

Candida is a great mimic. It can cause an amazing range of baffling symptoms, including chronic fatigue, pains, abdominal bloating, weight gain and even clinical depression. If left unchecked, it can also result in irritable bowel syndrome.

Worst of all, Candida can cause severe mental disturbance, so that the patient may be at risk of falling into the hands of a psychiatrist, who will not even consider this condition but will use powerful drugs and even maybe shock treatment (some still do this barbarous "therapy").

Such an unlucky patient would never get well because she needs an anti-fungal and inner environment approach, not a psychiatric disease approach.

By the way, although the condition mainly affects women, men are also at risk of developing Candidiasis.

I believe it is scandalous that conventional medicine still refuses to recognize Candida as a serious medical condition other than thrush. Yet it is known that Candida becomes a serious menace when the immune system is compromised. What conventional doctors don't see is just how much our immune systems are damaged by junk food, pesticides, heavy metal poisoning, emotional stress and medications.

Candida has now reached epidemic proportions because of the large amounts of sugar and refined carbohydrates we typically consume in our diets. This is one of the main causes. Other major causes are the widespread use of antibiotics, the contraceptive pill and HRT, which all increase your risk of developing a yeast overgrowth.

So What Is Candida?

You'll hear this term a lot. Let me warn you, it's not even that simple. But some cases are definitely Candida-based.

Candida albicans is a single-celled yeast (similar to fungus) that is just one of several hundred species of microorganisms living in your gut. Another species, Candida glabrata can also raise its ugly head.

Normally Candida poses no threat to your health, and is kept in check by beneficial gut bacteria but when the balance of your natural 'gut flora' becomes upset (because of poor diet, medication or prolonged stress), Candida can run riot throughout your body, causing generalized Candidiasis with disastrous results.

Classically this happens when you have been taking repeated or long-term antibiotics. Note that generalized Candida (throughout the body) is NOT the same as "systemic" Candida. That's much more serious, often fatal, and you will encounter a lot of disinformation on this point. Some of it, sad to say, from my old buddy William G. Crook, an early writer on this topic (now deceased). His otherwise marvelous book "The Yeast Connection" is a classic and remains in circulation today, long after Bill passed away.

The genus Candida and species C. albicans was first described by botanist Christine Marie Berkhout in her doctoral thesis at the University of Utrecht in 1923. Obsolete names for this genus include Mycotorula and Torulopsis. The species has also been known in the past as Monilia albicans and Oidium albicans.

The genus Candida covers about 150 different species, however, only a few are known to cause human infections: C. albicans is the most significant pathogenic species. Other Candida species pathogenic in humans include C. tropicalis, C. glabrata, C. krusei, C. parapsilosis, C. dubliniensis, and C. lusitaniae.

When people talk about "yeast infections", they really mean this group of organisms, not real yeast such as brewer's and baker's yeast (though these are relevant, and part of the problem, as we shall see).

Systemic Candida should be reserved for the terminal condition, often the cause of death in AIDS and cancer patients, where the immune system has collapsed so greatly that the blood and tissues are riddled with Candida and the body can't fight it off.

Used in this (proper) sense, systemic Candida is very like septicemia caused by a bacterium species. This too is often rapidly fatal.

Other Forms

It's true that Candida can spread and invade, without necessarily killing the victim.

The yeast can mutate from a single-celled organism to a thread-like 'mycelial' form, which penetrates your gut wall and enters your bloodstream. This makes your gut 'leaky', so that partly digested food molecules can enter your bloodstream and set off allergic reactions.

In your gut, Candida ferments sugary foods to produce carbon dioxide, which causes bloating and flatulence. It also produces alcohols and other complex chemicals that irritate the lining of your gut.

This has the effect of making your gut go into painful spasms and is less able to assimilate food, leading to constipation or diarrhea. These effects make Candida a major cause (although not the only one) of irritable bowel syndrome. As it spreads through your body, Candida also produces increasing quantities of toxic by-products, which can cause a host of physical and mental symptoms. There is a table of possible symptoms on page 26, that will help you decide if it might be your problem.

Because the symptoms of Candidiasis are so varied and vague, for years conventional medicine has largely put patient's symptoms down to hysteria or malingering. Even today, whilst Candida is acknowledged as the cause of thrush, many doctors continue to ignore the fact that candidiasis is a 'real' medical condition.

Unfortunately, I also see enthusiasts in holistic medicine diagnosing Candida at every turn. Most of this is wildly inaccurate because lists of symptoms like the one I have given here have many possible causes. The Candida symptoms list on page 26 is almost identical with the food and chemical allergy list and with the Lyme's list (real Lyme's or fibromyalgia)!

Really, these symptoms are simply those of a body overloaded with toxins and unable to self-correct or cope.

Confusion and Disinformation

I find it surprising, that even with a great deal of media attention to yeast infections, doctors' journals continue to ignore it. Candida is in and out of the news. For example, it gained notoriety in the UK when a pop star's wife was said to suffer from yeast infection.

This led to the public awareness of the condition. What was shocking was when the public watched her sickness worsen over the days, and it became clear that the treatment was more deadly than the disease.

As such, you can be excused for asking what the real facts are surrounding yeast infection. There is so much false information and general ignorance that it's a wonder anything is known about the condition at all.

Inside this book, I will attempt to summarize just what we do know about Candida so that you can fully understand everything you need to know. This is of course necessary in order to cure your current condition.

I also hope to put an end to some of the nonsense and falsehoods, spread by unqualified medical practitioners. It is a shame that these people spread untruths about yeast infections by claiming to be 'Candida experts'.

This is one the reasons that I decided to create this book.

The Internet makes it very easy for people to pose as having knowledge and information on a particular subject matter. Unfortunately kind hearted and trusting people get sucked into their trap.

The real problem that I have with these people is that their claims are not just false, they can also put people's health at risk. This is something that I am completely against.

The information that you will find in this book is all medically sound and based on proven principles from qualified, reputable doctors.

Perhaps you have seen the results of the treatment of some charlatans? For example, there have been women who fade away, getting skinnier and weaker because they obsessively avoid almost all foods. They won't eat sugars, starches, fruits (because of sugar), root vegetables (because of mold) or mushrooms (because they are similar to mold).

This causes long-term health problems and only happens because a fool has told them that such foods are dangerous. The real truth is that food is a significant part of the problem but not the majority of foods.

Misleading "Treatments"

A lot of the confusion about Candida comes from the fact that a number of widely circulated 'anti-Candida diets' do have beneficial effects. You may be someone who has read about such diets and perhaps even tried them.

It is really important to realize that there is a difference in removing a food causing an allergy and totally eradicating Candida. Oftentimes this is completely misunderstood by "experts" who believe they have found a miracle cure.

What actually occurs in these circumstances is that women remove a certain food group from their diet and miraculously recover. This happens because certain people are allergic to some foods in the first place. This creates the false impression that the patients had actually had Candida.

For example, there was a diet in Sweden that told patients to exclude dairy produce as part of an anti-Candida regime. There was also a naturopath in Britain that claimed 'no grains' was the way to a cure. There is absolutely no rationale for removing these food groups in the fight against Candida.

All they do is ensure that a great many people who are dairy or wheat allergic will 'miraculously' get better and are then convinced Candida was the problem.

There is another incorrect theory that has been circulating recently. It goes like this: once you have Candida, you're stuck with it.

Again, in these circumstances it is the amateur's fundamental lack of knowledge that causes the problems and misunderstandings. This leads to stories of people who are said to have had Candida for years.

The truth is that many sufferers of yeast infection are denied the full treatment that they need because the "expert" lacks the correct knowledge to diagnose it. Not only this, their amateur status prevents them from prescribing the proper anti-fungal drugs. This is a treatment that would enable people to overcome their condition much more rapidly.

There are even people today who suggest it is undesirable to take an anti-fungal medication because they are not able to properly eradicate the condition.

As you can see, there is a lot of bad information out there, which I will expose and clear up for you throughout this book.

What Causes Candida/Yeast Infections?

A Candida/yeast infection is a complex condition and it cannot be pinned down to a single cause. It can be triggered by more than one factor, which is why it is difficult to control. This is one of the reasons that research is still ongoing after many years, and why doctors find it very difficult to completely eradicate, even using prescription drugs.

The main causes of Candida/yeast syndrome are:

- Broad-spectrum antibiotics
- Lowered immunity
- Sugary, starchy diets (negative nutrition)
- Steroid drugs (including the oral contraceptive group)
- Other immune-compromising drugs (chemotherapy group)
- Prolonged illness (becoming rundown and debilitated)
- Stress (lowers the immune system)

ME cases also seem to get it very consistently. Any long-term debilitating illness may be accompanied by what we call 'opportunistic infections' (the yeast infection can take hold while the patient's resistance is low).

Oral sex, heavy smoking and wearing dentures are also sometimes suggested as risk factors.

Given time, the fungal stage of Candida can even penetrate throughout the bowel wall, passing into the bloodstream and through the body. Once this happens, it can cause depression, listlessness, extreme fatigue during the day, and a 'hung over' feeling in the morning. We call this Candidiasis, really "Candida illness" (not to be confused with "systemic Candida", which I have already explained is different and is far more serious).

One of the obvious results of Candida profusion may be thrush in the mouth or the vagina. The latter affects only women, of course, but men can get thrush on (and in) their penis. Thrush is easily seen as a white slimy paste spread over the membranes (Candida is from a Latin word, which means "pure white").

The important point, when considering how to eradicate this pest, is how to stop it coming back.

If you don't fix the inner environment or "terrain", the problem will just recur. If the patient is like a fertile garden for yeast weeds, they will grow and flourish at every opportunity. Sugar, for instance, feeds Candida like crazy. Yeasts ferment sugar and make alcohol. That's how they get their energy. That's how we get our wine and beer! You need to create a yeast desert inside your body (no, not a desert for humans; we would feel healthy and zestful).

There are a number of ways you can attempt to bring the inner environment back into balance. These multi-factor approaches are going to be discussed in the following pages. They are safer, more natural, much simpler and far more likely to work than just taking anti-fungal drugs or even garlic and iodine!

We shall be looking at all aspects of this process of cleaning up the inner "terrain". Pay particular attention to Quinton Marine Plasma (QMP) on page 84.

History Keeps Repeating

Many people have advocated the idea that the cause of yeast infection is a yeast-like organism that lives on starches and sugars and causes bowel disturbance. This idea is not new.

In fact, it seems to come back into fashion (in medical circles) every few decades and then lapses out of sight once again. The reason for this idea dates back to the 1980s, when some doctors became convinced they had found the causes of yeast infection. The problem arises as they are unable to find a workable proof that offers a satisfactory explanation. This casts doubt on the basis of the theory.

The success of anti-fungal drugs may have fed a myth. In some cases, anti-Candida therapeutic agents such as Nystatin seem to work only in very high doses (10 to 100 times the usual dose). This has led to the speculation that it may be helping by some other mechanism than just that of eradicating the yeast micro-organism; possible by blocking bowel permeability.

One thing is certain, there is virtually no correlation between Candida in the stool sample and the existence of the 'yeast syndrome'. Indeed, Candida albicans is rarely identified in specimens, despite its known very wide occurrence. This lack of correlation is disappointing but hardly surprising, especially if we are looking for the wrong culprit.

Could It Be Something Else?

It is certainly true that treatment directed towards this type of organism can be highly effective in selected individuals, so clearly a real phenomenon exists.

But that doesn't prove that Candida is to blame. In fact I'd like to set the debate alight with the claim that the culprit may not be Candida at all, or that Candida is only one of many potential suspects.

Other available flora that might be at work includes the ordinary yeasts of the genus Saccharomyces (food yeasts), certain species of E. Coli, Pseudammonas (pyruvate fermentation) and, most fascinating of all, Sarcina ventriculi. These all occur in our bodies and can ferment to make alcohol and other toxic compounds.

Historically, Sarcina is an important organism. In the old days, when surgeons operated in frock coats and quite often smoked cigars at the same time, once in a while they would literally blow up their patients. This happened as the alcoholic gases generated by Sarcina were released from the patient's stomach when cut open. At such time, the cigar would ignite the fumes and a fireball was the disastrous result.

It still happens today, though rarely, due to electrical diathermy equipment igniting explosive colonic gases.

These 'on-board breweries' are probably quite common. The late Dr Keith Eaton called my attention to the speculation that so-called 'spontaneous combustion' may be due to this microbe. Puzzling cases have been documented of human beings literally vanishing in a sheet of fire, for no apparent reason. Perhaps Sarcina, or some other organism, and its inflammable gaseous excreta could be to blame.

So from now on, through the rest of this book, remember when I say just "Candida" or "yeasts", I am really referring to a whole group of organisms that are capable of fermenting carbohydrates and will seize opportunities to invade little ecological niches within our bodies, caused by loss of friendly bacteria and/or dietary indiscretions; in fact any debilitating factor that compromises our ability to shrug them off.

There is no one strain of yeast or one strain of Candida.

The Classic "Mickey Finn"

Incidentally, just as Candida isn't the only contender for the role of pathogen, ordinary ethyl alcohol is not the only product of fermentation we seem to be dealing with.

In fact, many other products can be derived from the breakdown of sugars and starches, including short-chain fatty acids such as acetate, proprionate, succinate and butyrate, and other alcohols such as iso-propanol, butanol and 2, 3 – butylene glycol. Many of the chemicals now turn up in cosmetics and household goods, making the job of testing for significant levels a problem.

Further, if detoxification pathways are blocked due to overload, other unwanted metabolites are produced, such as epoxides, aldehydes and even chloral hydrate, ingredient of the classic 'Mickey Finn'.

Typically this chemical produces a tired and 'spacey' feeling. Here is at least part of the reason these patents can't take alcoholic drinks. Naturally, these by-products have a bad effect on the patient and most are quite toxic.

For treatment of this condition, all that is written about Candida is probably valid, at least until we know the truth about what we are dealing with. Anti-fungals usually help, but probiotics are more logical. Avoidance of fermentable sugars is important.

Paradoxically, antibiotics occasionally solve the problem; presumably when the culprit is a fermenting bacillus, such as Sarcina. Not many dogma thinkers have been willing to follow me into that territory but I assure you I have had desirable results when able to think this laterally!

The Chicago Restaurant Poisonings

On June 22, 1918, four people were arrested and over one hundred waiters taken into custody over the apparent widespread practice of poisoning by waiters in Chicago. Guests who tipped poorly were given "Mickey Finn powder" in their food or drinks.

Chemical analysis showed that it contained antimony and potassium tartrate, known to cause headaches, dizziness, depression, and vomiting and can be lethal in large quantities. Incredibly, somebody was manufacturing and selling packets of the chemical cocktail specifically for spiteful waiters. Talk about finding a sales niche!

Future Research
Identification of Yeast Mating Habits Opens New Doors to Candida Research

The discovery of mating behavior in the yeast Candida albicans was published in the 2000 issue of the journal Science.

Candida was long thought to reproduce only by splitting itself in half. The new study, supported by the National Institute of Allergy and Infectious Diseases (NIAID), provide new opportunities for scientists to better understand the diseases caused by this fungus.

We now know it does a simple version of sexual reproduction, that is: two different organisms getting together and swapping genes, resulting in a new "offspring".

Unlike baker's yeast, where the genetic systems and mating have been extensively analyzed in the laboratory, C. albicans has proven very private in its sex life till recently!

Now we have caught examples of it mating!

This discovery promises to accelerate research into the fungus and enable researchers to more quickly understand its biology and identify new drug targets.

Who Was Mickey Finn?

The Mickey Finn is most likely named for the manager and bartender of a Chicago restaurant, which operated from 1896 to 1903 in the city's South Loop neighborhood on South State Street.

He was accused of using knockout drops to incapacitate and rob some of his customers. Finn's saloon was ordered closed on December 16, 1903.

The term "Mickey Finn" first appeared in the Oxford English Dictionary in 1915, twelve years after his trial, lending credence to this theory of the origination of the phrase.

Before his days as a saloon proprietor, Mickey Finn was known as a pickpocket and thief who often preyed on drunken bar patrons. The act of serving a Mickey Finn Special was a coordinated robbery orchestrated by Finn. First, Finn or one of his employees, which included "house girls", would slip a drug (chloral hydrate) in the unsuspecting patron's drink. The incapacitated patron would be escorted or carried into a back room by one of Finn's associates who would then rob the victim and dump him in an alley.

The finding has important implications beyond simplifying Candida research. Scientists have shown that in another disease-causing organism, Cryptococcus, one mating type is much more virulent than the other. If this is true for C. albicans it opens up a new approach to therapeutics.

The researchers expect their discovery to accelerate studies on how the fungus adapts to different environments and how it evades the body's defense mechanisms.

CHAPTER 1

Background To The Candida Story

Dr C. Orian Truss MD of Birmingham, Alabama, was the first person since the 1930s to propose the Candida hypothesis (1978 paper). Dr. Truss was a psychiatrist and has a special interest in clinical ecology.

What he revealed brought new light to the problem that many people had been suffering with. After Dr. Truss, another doctor by the name of William G. Crook MD took this work further.

Crook was the man who really popularized the Candida hypotheses. This has now become known as the 'the yeast connection', which was the name used in his book.

Since that time, the whole theory seems to have gripped the public's imagination and clinical ecologists have been keen to deal with the existence of the problem. This has led to far more research and discovery so that now we know the enormous benefits to be gained from tackling it vigorously.

There are health gains to be made by following an anti-Candida program, taking anti-fungal drugs and excluding sugar and yeast foods from one's diet. Yet Truss's idea is no more than a theory.

The one valid complaint that members of the medical profession have against clinical ecologists is the time that is takes them to back up the ideas with research.

In fact, it has now been over 25 years since Truss's innovative papers. This should have been enough time to carry out many in depth studies that would validate his claims. Yet such studies are still not in existence. This is despite the fact that the problem has been around a very long time.

As you know, a catalogue of startling recoveries does not constitute scientific study. We may be getting the right results for the wrong reason.

Earlier Little Known History

During my research over the decades, I found a Dr. Turner anticipated Truss's ideas almost 70 years earlier. Turner presented a paper on what he called 'intestinal germ carbohydrate fermentation' (proceedings of the Royal Society of Medicine Symposium of Intestinal Toxaemia, 1911).

Later, in 1931 Hurst was in his footsteps, and wrote about 'intestinal carbohydrate dyspepsia'. In the 1930s and 1940s this dyspepsia was being treated with Lactobacillus acidophilus, B vitamin supplements and a low-starch diet (remarkably like modern anti-Candida treatments except that legumes are no longer banned, as they were at that time).

Since that time, medical literature has tried to define the patient-type who suffers with this syndrome.

There was a major text on gastroenterology during 1976. This described victims as 'Essentially unhappy people . . . any suggested panacea or therapeutic straw is grasped . . . no regime is too severe and no program too difficult . . . with the tenacity of the faithful, they grope their way from one practitioner to the next in the search for a permanently successful remedy.'

I believe this disparaging description shows an appalling weakness by certain doctors for blaming any patient they cannot help.

The 'problem patient' attitude was probably what sank the "Candida" or yeast condition in the 1950s. During this time, the psychosomatic theory of disease was enjoying a great revival. The tendency was to dismiss all patients with vague, ill-defined symptoms as psychiatric cases. Unlike today, there were no physical findings to disprove the psychiatric label and so it stuck. It's still with us, to a large degree.

What Is Candida Or Yeast Infection?

As I will explain later, "Candida" is really just an umbrella name for overgrowth organisms which may include Candida albicans but is certainly not the only culprit. Regular food yeasts (the saccharomyces) are quite capable of producing all the symptoms. Some of this comes from bread and alcoholic drinks but there are plenty of yeasts on the skin of foods and also molds which settle from the atmosphere.

Candida and other yeast-like organisms are normally found on our bodies and in the large bowel. If we are healthy it poses little threat. But if it is given a special advantage, as with today's rubbish diets, or our immune systems are compromised, it can proliferate and become troublesome or even dangerous.

The worst provocation factor of all is antibiotics. The indiscriminate use of these substances, especially the so-called broad spectrum kind (such as tetracycline or amoxicillin), leads to loss of normal healthy bacteria that can and should exist on and within our bodies. Once these friendly flora are removed, then Candida can assert itself without competition and it switches to a very aggressive mode of growth.

Depressed Immune Function

Candida proliferation is caused mainly by a compromised immune system, which in turn may be due to stress, poor nutrition, lack of exercise or adequate rest, pollution, smoking, alcohol consumption, HIV infection, cyto-toxic cancer therapy, and or steroid therapy.

The immune system is one of the guardians of a balanced floral community. It ensures that no one organism dominates the scene. When the immune system gets compromised then aggressive organisms such as Candida albicans tend to take over and overgrow their rightful place in the floral community.

Many women suffering from chronic vaginal Candidiasis are caught in the "Candida Vicious Cycle" which involves immune suppression and antibiotic use.

Here is the cycle explained in more detail:

- The stress of modern living causes depressed immune function.
- Depressed immune function results in bacterial infections requiring antibiotics.
- The antibiotics disturb the floral balance.
- With bacterial neighbors absent and a depleted immune function in place, Candida albicans proliferates.

- To worsen the situation, Candida albicans produces immune suppressive substances. The additionally depressed immune function leaves the patient more vulnerable to bacterial infection.
- Additional antibiotics are required.
- Around and around the cycle goes.

Vaginal thrush has a very big impact on the daily lives of many women. During one study of 200 women, they all stated that allopathic treatment with creams and pessaries previously undertaken only brought short-term relief and did not end the cycle. The anti-fungal creams only had an effect when applied and did nothing to insure the condition would not return. This cycle is widely recognized, and as of yet, there is no effective treatment available aimed at ending it.

The real cure or eradication of Candida and yeast infections is a much wider issue, as we shall see. To merely give symptomatic relief, by addressing only the localized problem, is to fail to strike at the real cause of the condition and so remedy it.

Poor Diet Is A Problem

A diet that is high in carbohydrates and toxic foods (especially sugar) affects the biochemical processes within the cells. This creates problems in digestion and also prevents the natural toxic elimination process from working, as it should.

The foods that cause this are those highly processed, unnatural foods that are so common today. You will see later in the book how a change in diet can have significant improvements in your health. If your diet is currently low in fresh fruit and vegetables then you need to change your diet.

Here's why. The conditions you are creating inside your body are actually feeding the growth of Candida (on a poor diet). Candida thrives on refined carbohydrates such as sugar, white flour and white rice.

This is a problem that can be made even worse if you are deficient in vital nutrients. The ideal conditions for the overgrowth of Candida are the supply of food (listed above) and a nutritional deficiency.

If you have poor nutrition then you are giving Candida the perfect breeding ground. Your body needs about forty essential vitamins, minerals and nutrients to let the cells in your body function, as they should. This is also needed in order that you remain in good health.

As these nutrients and minerals come from your diet, you need to make good food choices. The body is not able to produce the essential minerals and nutrients itself, so if your diet is poor, you are in effect starving your body.

The more processed foods that you eat, the less effective your immune system will be. This is because your immune system relies on the nutrients that you give it in order to function at its best. When your immune system is weak, the overgrowth of Candida is much more likely, and far easier to get out of control.

The over-acidic nature of the digestive system is another major factor in the cause of yeast infection. This is usually because of a highly acidic diet. When a highly acid diet is used, the blood becomes thick which is an ideal environment for Candida growth.

As you will see in a later chapter, the key to expelling Candida is to optimize your immune system. When this is achieved, it really helps to expel yeasts and bacteria. If your digestive system becomes sluggish, then undigested food and rotten food particles in the blood stream and digestive tract will increase the symptoms and encourage Candida overgrowth.

Why Sugar Is A Double Whammy

Sugar is fermentable. That's how yeasts create energy from foodstuffs. If you eat foods containing sugar, you are in effect feeding the Candida. It FEASTS on cookies, candies and muffins!

But there is a second reason why sugary foods are disastrous. Sugar suppresses the immune system. Scientific studies have shown clearly that any significant sugar intake stuns white blood cells for up to 6 hours after eating. This is the last thing you need.

Suppressed immunity is one of the major reasons that Candida and yeasts get started.

Antibiotics And Prescription Drugs

In 1953 Dr Orian Truss discovered the devastating effects of antibiotics in an Alabama (USA) hospital. During a hospital round, Truss was intrigued by a gaunt, apparently elderly man who was obviously dying.

However, the patient was only in his forties and had only been in hospital for four months. In that time, no specialist had been able to make a diagnosis. Out of curiosity Truss asked the patient when be was last completely well.

The man answered that he had been well until he had cut his finger six months earlier. He had received antibiotics for this. Shortly afterwards he developed diarrhea and his health deteriorated.

Truss had noted before how antibiotics cause diarrhea. It was known that Candida was opportunistic and thrived in debilitated patients, but now Truss wondered if it might not be the other way round, that Candida actually caused the debilitated condition.

He had read that potassium Iodide solution could be used to treat Candida infestation of the blood. So he put the patient on six to eight drops of Lugol's solution four times a day and soon the patient was completely well.

Soon afterwards he had a female patient with a stuffy nose, a throbbing headache, vaginitis and severe depression. To his amazement all her problems immediately cleared with Candida treatment.

Some time later he saw a female patient who had been schizophrenic for six years with hundreds of electroshock treatments and massive drug dosages. He started treating the woman for sinus allergies with a Candida neutralization vaccine. Soon she had recovered mentally and physically, and remained well.

From then on he treated his patients against Candida at the slightest indication of its presence. Many of his patients made remarkable recoveries from most unusual conditions including menstrual problems, hyperactivity, learning disabilities, autism, multiple sclerosis and auto-immune diseases such as Crohn's disease and lupus erythematosus.

Every experienced naturopath can relate similar success stories. Ironically, antibiotics are usually not necessary in the first place. In a few percent of the cases in which they are necessary, their serious after effects could easily be avoided using fungicides and lactobacilli.

Many people doubt the effectiveness of natural therapies against apparently serious infections, but my experience leads me to believe that natural therapies are frequently more effective, without causing the repeated and chronic infections seen after antibiotics. I have seen patients who have been unsuccessful on long-term antibiotic treatment recover within days or weeks with natural therapies.

In chapter 4, I devote the entire chapter to the discussion of natural remedies and they can be applied when yeast infection is present.

Weakened Immune System
The body becomes very vulnerable when the immune system is weakened. This occurs due to many factors such as nutritional deficiency, stress, lack of sleep, the use of drugs (prescription and otherwise), high toxic buildup (viruses, heavy metal, chemicals, parasite, bacteria).

When the immune system is weak, the body cannot defend itself as it should and the process of Candida overgrowth can take over.

As such, pathological Candida albicans proliferation is common in the immune suppressed. For example, AIDS patients and those on immunosupressive drug regimes are two notable examples.

However, the vast majority of patients suffering from chronic vaginal Candida albicans proliferations (Thrush) do not fall into either of these categories. They are women with apparently normal immune systems, women that have fallen into what is often described as the "Candida Vicious Cycle". Bad diet and lifestyle is the usual precipitating factor to look for.

Sexual Activity

Yeast infection can be contagious and passed during sexual activity. This is especially true in the case of a yeast infection in the vaginal or penis area. Of course, using protection and being cautious is a very important step in preventing the spread of yeast infection.

It is important when treating a woman for vaginal thrush to also treat her male partner. Otherwise we get into what we call "ping pong" infections: he gives it to her and she gives it to him, back and forth.

By the way, I had better add in this liberated age that I have encountered lesbian couples where one partner had oral thrush and the other vaginal thrush. I expect the same phenomenon can affect male homosexuals, though I have no experience of this.

Chronic Nasal Congestion
In the August 1998 issue of the Annals of Allergy, Asthma, and Immunology, Brazilian researchers reported that many women with recurrent vaginal Candida were also prone to perennial allergic rhinitis (chronic nasal congestion). The condition is designated as "recurrent" if at least four episodes occur within 12 months.

Researchers compared the incidence of allergic diseases in two groups of women over the course of 28 months. In the first group were 95 healthy women with normal immune systems; all had recurrent vaginal Candidiasis and were referred to a private allergy practice. The second group consisted of 100 women who visited the same allergy practice; none suffered from recurrent vaginal candidiasis. C

Previous research has hinted at a link between nasal allergies and chronic or recurring vaginal candidiasis. The findings of the current study make the point in a more definitive way, concluding that the nasal allergies may in fact be a predisposing factor for the vaginal condition.

In contrast to the control group, women with recurrent vaginal Candidiasis had a high relative incidence of skin tests positive to inhalant allergens and to C. albicans. There was no correlation to asthma; only allergic nasal symptoms.

Symptoms And Self-Assessment

This section is going to present you with the most common symptoms so that you can conduct a self-assessment. Check yourself and you decide whether you have a Candida/yeast problem; don't rely on your health care practitioner, who may not even believe in this disease.

Please note that it is extremely important to obtain an accurate diagnosis before trying to find a cure. Many diseases and conditions share common symptoms: if you treat yourself for the wrong illness or a specific symptom of a complex disease, you may delay legitimate treatment of a serious underlying problem. In other words, the greatest danger in self-treatment may be self-diagnosis.

But most patients have no choice but to try, since conventional help has failed them. Here are symptoms to guide you in making a decision.

If many of the symptoms and factors listed below apply to you, it is likely that you're suffering from Candida:

- Bloating and discomfort, especially after meals.
- Griping pains in your lower abdomen.
- Constipation or diarrhea.
- Fatigue or muscle weakness.
- Muscle or joint pains, or arthritis.
- 'Brain fog', feelings of unreality or memory loss.
- Thrush, athlete's foot, ringworm or fungal infection of your nails.
- Urinary tract infection or vaginal discharge.
- Depression or tearfulness.
- 'Low' immune system and frequent infections.
- Sensitivities to foods, tobacco smoke, chemical odors or perfume.
- Cravings for sugar, bread or alcohol.
- Symptoms worse on damp, muggy days or in damp, moldy places.

This list is not exhaustive, meaning possible symptoms are not confined to those on this list. Any complex, chronic and baffling symptom should arouse a suspicion of hidden chronic infection. Candida and yeast are often overlooked as candidates for this.

Warning: all lists such as this contain symptoms that could have many other causes. It's the overall picture that counts.

Online Yeast Questionnaire(s)

You can take an on-line yeast questionnaire, based on the writings of my late friend William G. Crook MD: http://www.jigsawhealth.com/testing_candida.aspx

There is also an alternative assessment test for children: http://www.jigsawhealth.com/testing_children.aspx

The Awesome Foursome!

Over the years, I have been able to identify certain critical symptoms that help confirm the problem of Candida. I started with the "terrible trio":

1. bloating
2. sugar cravings
3. alcohol intolerance

If these three are present in a patient, I could presumptively diagnose Candida with a good degree of accuracy. 2 out of three was probable, too.

In time I learned to add chemical sensitivity. So now I call it my "awesome foursome"!

It is just a joke term but it helps patients to remember what they are up against and so is a useful mnemonic.

One thing is certain; there is virtually no correlation between Candida in a stool sample and the existence of the 'yeast syndrome'. Indeed, Candida albicans is rarely identified in specimens, despite its known very wide occurrence.

Female Yeast Symptoms

Vulvitis (inflammation of the vulva) and vaginal pain, itching or dryness can soon drive you to despair, especially when it makes having sex difficult or even impossible. Of course, this can place a huge strain on your relationship.

There are three common types of vaginal irritation:

• Dryness
• Vestibulitis
• Deep vaginitis

Vaginal dryness often occurs during the menopause when estrogen production decreases. This has the effect of reducing lubricating secretions, causing soreness or itching and pain during intercourse. But it can affect younger women, when arousal is limited.

Vestibulitis is extreme sensitivity or inflammation around the entrance of the vagina. Although its cause is unknown, it can sometimes be triggered by a reaction to chemicals in soaps, talcum powder or deodorant. As such, make sure you avoid these if you're diagnosed with the condition.

The third type of vaginal infection is vaginitis. This is a burning or itching sensation that occurs deeper inside the vagina, which is often accompanied by a heavy or abnormal discharge. Yellowish-greenish and smelly discharge is not usually associated with Candida and means a different organism is likely (Trichomonas, for example). The characteristic thrush discharge is white, thick, almost cheesy, and intensely itchy. It may have a yeasty odor.

There is little mistaking it, once encountered.

It is important to note that there are some normal discharges during the menstrual cycle. These are also pale yellow/creamy in color and appear with a mucus-like thickness.

[MORE SYMPTOMS OVER THE PAGE]

Localized vaginal yeast infection symptoms:

- White and abnormal discharge from the vagina
- Itching and irritation – including burning in the vagina
- Pain during sexual intercourse
- Pain during urination
- Inflammatory redness in the perineum area
- Over sensitivity and irritation of the pubic hair follicles

More Severe Symptoms That May Be Encountered:

- Pain during urination
- General fatigue and lethargy
- Severe swelling of the vagina characterized by a swollen anus and purple color of the vulva.
- Walking difficulties
- Bleeding and swelling of hemorrhoid veins
- Pain during sexual intercourse
- Painful skin cracks because of severe dryness in the vagina area

Yeast Infections Of The Penis

I have already referred to the fact that yeast can affect males. In men infections of the male penis are commonly associated with symptoms such as redness or a rash. Sometimes these symptoms are accompanied by painful (burning) sensation with urination.

Uncircumcised men are able to carry the organism more closely disguised and sheltered from hygiene and the natural immune barriers protections present on all skin. Personal care thus becomes paramount, out of decency and concern for one's sexual partner.

Oral Thrush Symptoms

Oral thrush yeast infections are also associated with certain symptoms. Commonly, small cream colored, white, or yellow spots are present. Typically the spots are located on the tongue and back of the mouth. The spots are commonly painless; however, if these spots are scraped off, bleeding is typical. Thrush is also associated with an uncomfortable sensation of burning of the throat and mouth.

Fatigue

You should know that fatigue is very common when someone is suffering from Candidiasis, yeast and mold problems. Besides this, depression and changes in mood are also particularly prominent.

While the list above is very useful, it is also important to realize that lists of symptoms are not reliable guides to Candida infection or any other mold problem. Many lists give symptoms that are typical of a food allergy, ME (fibromyalgia) and many other states. These simply reflect a body under stress and not some specific condition.

Learning Difficulties

There is clear emerging evidence that yeast infections can affect schooling. [Yeast can Affect Behavior and Learning, William G. Crook Intervention in School and Clinic.1984; 19: 517-526]

Candida is likely to be passed on to the baby if its mother has thrush during pregnancy, resulting in problems appearing after just a few weeks.

Severe diaper rash, rectal rashes or infections, rashes in the genital area, and colic are the most common symptoms in babies. Thrush, general skin rashes, infections of the ear, nose, & throat, gas, diarrhea or constipation are all possible symptoms.

Other kids develop Candida after receiving lots of antibiotics

Kids' diets these days are pretty awful too, loaded with candies and sodas.

Candida is often a major factor in ADD, ADHD and behavioural problems. It gets mixed in with food allergic difficulties and also chemical sensitivity. Just as adults can experience fatigue and depression, kids afflicted by symptoms like these don't have a chance at school. They are "learning impaired" before they start!

If your child is affected (see questionnaire referred to on page 27), you need to implement all the advice in this book.

Can A Yeast Infection Be Life Threatening?

Typically, yeast infections are not life threatening. However, if a lack of proper and prompt treatment leads to the development of certain complications, then those things can be life threatening (if certain circumstances are met).

The severity of the yeast infection is dependent upon many individual factors. The most important factor is the strength and health of the immune system.

Individuals with weakened/compromised immune systems must take all Candida yeast infections seriously. The presence of a yeast infection may also be a sign of further decreases in immune system function. So it becomes a vicious circle, which is why we have such a problem here: lowered immune competence leads to yeast and Candida overgrowth, which then further suppresses the immune system, so more overgrowth occurs.

It can be difficult to break this vicious circle but it is important to do so.

Occasionally, Candida gets completely out of control and floods the blood stream. We call this systemic Candida and it can threaten life. It may be the final stage of a terminal disease, such as AIDS or cancer. Note that both of these conditions reflect a poorly functioning immune system (cancer patients taking chemo or radiotherapy suffer a disastrous loss of immune competence).

Diagnostic Laboratory Testing

Try to work with a practitioner with some knowledge of this condition. For more details on finding a liberal and knowledgeable doctor in your area, contact www.acam.org (USA) and The British Institute For Allergy And Environment therapy, Llangwyryfon, Aberystwyth, Ceredigion SY23 4EY Tel: 01974 241376 Fax: 01974 241795 www.allergy.org.uk

Almost all territories have a listing of such alternative practitioners. They will be able to help you with licensed tests and treatment. But stay away from lists of allergists and immunologists. They are the closed-minded set who don't believe much in alternative medicine; they prefer seasonal shots for allergies and steroids or antihistamines. Their knowledge of Candida is sparse to non-existent.

The first step in healing this condition is to get diagnosed. This is easier said than done since many mainstream doctors don't recognize Candida as a serious and debilitating disease. This leads many doctors to write its symptoms off as thrush or urinary tract infection.

The diagnosis issues also come from the lack of a suitable diagnostic test to show whether or not a patient has Candida. Some practitioners use applied kinesiology techniques but this is hardly acceptable to the medical community. Until a proper test is created and used as standard, the doctors need to rely heavily on taking a careful patient history, while being very careful to observe symptoms typical of those outlined above.

Many people are too embarrassed to see a doctor but you must see the gynecologist and discuss your yeast infection with them. If you see that you have many of the symptoms listed in the previous section then you need to make an appointment right away.

Your doctor will first examine the vulva and vagina area that is suspected to have the yeast infection. They will take a swab sample, which will then be sent to the lab so that it can be analyzed. This will let you know whether you have other types of infections besides the vaginal yeast infection.

It is a good idea to talk to your doctor about your concerns, feelings and symptoms. This will let the doctor know what you have been experiencing and let them understand the severity of the condition you are suffering from. This will also let them determine the best course of action for your specific needs. Obviously this dialogue works best if you have an understanding and well informed doctor.

Current tests that will help future diagnosis

Researchers have tried to establish a valid gut fermentation test. The idea is to take a resting blood alcohol level and then repeat the test some hours after a sugary feed. If alcohol appears in the blood this would suggest that fermentation is going on. But it doesn't tell us what is doing the fermenting. Candida can certainly ferment sugars. But so can ordinary food yeasts, which are present in out gut.

A likely improvement is to look for a wider range of fermentation products. Try to find a lab which is testing for short-chain fatty acids such as acetate, proprionate, succinate and butyrate, and for other alcohols such as iso-propanol, butanol and 2,3-butylene glycol.

Specific yeast/fungal markers include: Citramalic (methylmalic) acid, 5-hydroxymethyl-2-furoic acid, 3-oxoglutaric acid, Furan-2, 5-dicarboxylic acid, Furancarbonylglycine, Tartaric acid (hydroxymalic acid), Arabinose, Carboxycitric acid;

The advantage of these newer tests is that you don't need 'before' and 'after' samples, so it is easier to do.

The Organic Acids Test (OAT)

This is a refined version of the above testing modality, developed by the Great Plains Laboratory in Lenexa, Kansas, is the Organic Acids Test. It can be carried out on urine, which is more convenient than a blood sample for most people.

For chiros and other practitioners, it's good to know it has several CPT codes: 82507 82570 83150 83497 83605 83921*56 84210 84585

The Organic Acids Test (OAT) provides a metabolic "snapshot" based on those products the body discarded during urination. These small organic acid molecules are byproducts of human cellular activity, the digestion of foods, and the life cycles of gastrointestinal flora. Organic acids in urine may be toxic at certain levels or may simply be "markers" of metabolic pathways.

One distinction that makes The Great Plains Laboratory, Inc. OAT test so popular is the ability of this profile to reliably detect the overgrowth of yeast and bacteria species commonly missed by conventional culture methods. Metabolites of yeast or gastrointestinal bacteria appear against the background of normal human metabolites and provide a real-time assessment of yeast and bacterial activity. These organisms can produce or exacerbate symptoms in many conditions and often affect other metabolic processes assessed in the OAT.

Additional pathways of interest include products of carbohydrate digestion, mitochondrial function which produces most cellular energy, many vitamin levels, neurotransmitter metabolites, fatty acid oxidation abnormalities or ketosis, oxalate levels, and inborn errors of metabolism.

The test includes:
1. Yeast/fungal metabolites
2. Bacterial metabolites

3. B-vitamin deficiencies
4. Antioxidant deficiencies
5. Inborn errors of metabolism
6. Oxalate-related metabolites
7. Exposure to toluene solvent
8. Neurotransmitter metabolites
9. Indicators of possible diabetic conditions
10. Citric acid (Krebs) cycle metabolites
11. Clostridia overgrowth
12. Glycolysis metabolites
13. Fatty acid oxidation abnormalities
14. Amino acid metabolites
15. Pyrimidines

You will see this is a very comprehensive test and useful for anyone with chronic disease conditions. A total of 65 compounds are tested. This will set you back $250- 300 but is worth it.

You can download their comprehensive brochure here (which will supply good information, whatever country you live it):

http://www.greatplainslaboratory.com/home/eng/brochures/Organic%20Acids%20Test.pdf

Contact details:
Great Plains Laboratory
11813 W 77th St
Lenexa, KS 66214-1457
(913) 341-8949

Antibody Testing
There is some dispute over the subject of a Candida antibody test. Antibodies may be detected but that doesn't prove Candida is the problem; only that it has been a source of immune activity in the past.

ELIA immune-assay is very sensitive but that often means false positives.

Single testing is worthless. You need a test of several Candida immune complexes (IgA, IgG and IgM at least).

Immuno-Sciences Lab in Beverly Hills offers this kind of testing but at the time of writing their website was down, labeled "under construction".

Better turn instead to: Genova Diagnostics (Ashville, North Carolina) and Genova Diagnostics in New Maldeen, UK (for Europe). www.genovadiagnostics.com and www.gdx.uk.net respectively)

Genova Diagnostics
63 Zillicoa Street
Asheville, NC 28803
USA
Local Telephone: +(1) 828-253-0621

Practitioner Support Department
Monday through Friday 9 a.m. until 5.30 p.m. except for bank holidays
Telephone: + 44 (0) 208 336 7750 Fax: + 44 (0) 208 336 7751
Online: Please use our Practitioner Support Contact Form
Accounts Receivable Business Office

Genova Diagnostics Europe
Parkgate House
356 West Barnes Lane
New Malden
Surrey, KT3 6NB
Monday through Friday 9 a.m. until 5.30 p.m. except for bank holidays
Telephone: + 44 (0) 208 336 7759 Fax: + 44 (0) 208 336 7751
24hr Automated Kit Order Line: +44 (0) 208 336 7754
Kit Dispatch Department: +44 (0) 208 336 7763
Fax kit orders: 020 8336 7751

Online: They have a Kit Orders Contact Form [http://www.gdx.uk.net/index.php?option=com_chronocontact&chronoformname=accounts_receivable_contact_form&Itemid=114]

Pan-Fungal Panel (PFP)

Modern PCR (polymerase chain reaction) testing can now provide rapid, sensitive and specific detection of a wide variety of pathogens sometimes found in or causing difficult-to-diagnose conditions.

PCR can be used to identify the presence of seemingly hidden disease-causing viruses and/or bacteria and is capable of differentiating even closely-related organisms. It can be used to identify genetic markers that are associated with susceptibility or resistance to certain diseases, including diseases as diverse as diabetes, arthritis, cancer or allergies.

US Biotek Laboratories is one of the leading labs offering PCR testing. They have many disease panels available which will screen for suspected organisms in such cases, including a pan-fungal panel. US Biotek Laboratories claims unparallelled accuracy in determining the presence of specific microbial pathogens that could be complicating your health.

Therapeutic Trial
At the end of the day, we may rely on what is called a "therapeutic trial". That is, we give the patient the appropriate treatment and, if it works, we infer he or she must have had the disease.

It sounds crude but a lot of supposedly scientific medicine is done this way! It's still the best approach for Candida/yeast.

If I Have Thrush, Should I Be Worried?

Thrush is easily managed in healthy children and adults. But it can be a more serious problem if you have a weakened immune system.

Should I see a doctor for thrush?

If you are an otherwise healthy adult or child, you could try taking care of it on your own first. If it doesn't go away, thrush could be a symptom of a more serious problem that is weakening your immune system. You ought to see your doctor if your thrush persists.

Yeast Infection Complications

Yeast infections can be cause for specific complications that can be life threatening. The presence of certain symptoms including nausea/vomiting, vaginal discharge accompanied with abdominal pain, fever and chills should be reported to a physician.

These symptoms are common with certain conditions such as pelvic inflammatory disease, kidney infections, and appendicitis. These conditions require prompt hospital treatments.

Oral thrush can also have specific complications. If the thrush interferes with drinking or eating for extended periods of time, hospitalization may be necessary for other treatments and to re-establish fluid levels within the body.

It is not common for Candida skin infections to require hospitalization. However, recurring cases should be reported to a physician. The most aggressive and life threatening form of a Candidiasis infection is that of systemic Candidiasis.

Systemic Candidiasis

It is possible for yeast infections (Candidiasis) to become a systemic condition upon entering the bloodstream. This is most commonly associated with the presence of a compromised/weakened immune system. Systemic Candidiasis is caused by infection of the Candida fungus growth within internal organs or the bloodstream. Systemic Candidiasis can be life threatening without prompt investigation and treatment.

This is NOT the same a generalized Candida. It is closer in line to septicemia caused by bacteria.

Toxicity & Leaky Gut Syndrome

Candida is able to ferment and release alcohols from sugars in food. To many people these alcohols are quite allergenic. There have been several celebrated cases in which individuals who were guilty of driving under the influence of alcohol were able to show they had not been drinking but that they did have significant infections with Candida and so escaped the laws.

Remember Candida is a yeast, related to molds, and these organisms themselves are also often quite toxic and may be highly allergenic in their own right.

But the real problem is that Candida also appears able to generate food and chemical sensitivities. Increase in food intolerance has been blamed on damage to the gut wall. Like many yeasts and fungi, Candida has a vegetative from, which grows out small threads or hyphae into the surrounding cells.

It has been hypothesized that these hyphae may provide channels through which the products of digestion escape prematurely into the bloodstream. This means that food substances have not been broken down fully and are thus still biochemically 'wheat', 'pork' etc.

If this were so we would certainly expect trouble form allergies, so the supposition fits with the observed facts. But please remember, it is only another theory. It sounds good but may be totally wrong. Clinical ecologists call it the 'leaky gut syndrome'.

Some workers speak of "systemic Candida" but they are mistaken in what that means; systemic Candida is serious and often the final stage of a fatal disease.

They are really referring to a generalized illness "Candidiasis". A patient can feel sick all over without it implying that the organism is everywhere in the body. Candida releases toxins, as many microbes do, and it is these toxins that lead to widespread unpleasant symptoms.

It is important to note that Candida is never found in the blood stream in these cases. Only when the person is fatally ill can it usually be found in the blood, in the last stages of body overwhelm.

Immuno-assay showing possible raised antibodies to Candida albicans may occur. But, for the same reason, does not really prove that the organism has gone systemic, only that antibodies appear in the blood and therefore circulate widely.

In Summary: The Signs Of Candida/Yeast Overgrowth?

As a summary to this chapter, I think it is important to address this question again. If many of the symptoms and factors listed below apply to you, it is likely that you're suffering from candidiasis:

- Bloating and discomfort, especially after meals.
- Griping pains in your lower abdomen.
- Constipation or diarrhea.
- Fatigue or muscle weakness.
- Muscle or joint pains, or arthritis.
- 'Brain fog', feelings of unreality or memory loss.
- Thrush, athlete's foot, ringworm or fungal infection of your nails.
- Urinary tract infection or vaginal discharge.
- Depression or tearfulness.
- 'Low' immune system and frequent infections.
- Sensitivities to foods, tobacco smoke, chemical odors or perfume.
- Antibiotics taken for more than one month or more than four times within 12 months.
- Prednisolone or other steroid drugs taken for more than two weeks.
- Anti-ulcer drugs (e.g. Zantac, Tagamet) taken for more than two months.
- Birth control pill or hormone replacement therapy for more than two years.
- Cravings for sugar, bread or alcohol.
- Symptoms worse on damp, muggy days or in damp, moldy places.

CHAPTER 2

Molds and Mycotoxins

Many Candida and yeast patients notice a strong sensitivity to molds too. These are somewhat related biologically. This chapter will cover molds and mycotoxins, which is very important to know and understand. It will also deal with the link between these two things and yeast and Candida.

These things can lead to a number of related allergies, intolerance and toxicity problems. All of them are connected by the category of organisms in the group. Molds, fungi and yeast are considered neither animal nor vegetable but something in between.

The organisms of the fungal lineage include:

- Mushrooms
- Rusts
- Smuts
- Puffballs
- Truffles
- Morels
- Molds
- Yeasts
- As well as many less well-known organisms.

About 70,000 species of fungi have been described at present. However some estimates of the total number suggest that more than 1.5 million species may exist.

The fungi constitute an independent group equal in rank to that of plants and animals. They share with animals the ability to export hydrolytic enzymes that break down biological substances, which can be absorbed for nutrition. They don't need a stomach; we call this external digestion.

You may have noticed how molds can attack stale food or a dead animal corpse. The mold lives in and on the decaying substance and breaks it down.

Paul Stametz has shown us that molds are capable of breaking down even the worst environmental pollutants and turning them into safe, nutritious and friendly food stuff for plants and animals.

See the inspiring TED video on this web page: http://www.living-wisely.com/mycelium-mold-invented-the-internet/

Molds Are A Serious Health Problem

More worldwide food crops are lost to mold than any other single cause. However, we actually need molds to rot away rubbish and dead matter. Along with certain bacteria, molds clean up organic waste and stop the planet becoming a gigantic garbage heap. As such, you can see that we have an uneasy relationship with them.

Fungi include mushrooms, molds and yeasts. They may invade human tissues causing things such as skin infections or Candidiasis of the bowel.

Fungi can also cause direct or indirect toxic effects via secreted poisons called mycotoxins. These substances are often powerful immuno-suppressants and thus further reduce the individual's resistance, not only to mold infections but also to bacteria and viruses.

A number of clinical conditions are caused by mold infections, apart from the more obvious athlete's foot and ringworm. These include farmer's lung (caused by moldy hay), cheesewasher's lung (from a strain of penicillin) and bagassosis, a condition that affects those working with sugar cane infected with molds (bagasse is the remains of the treated cane plant, after sugar extraction).

We are all exposed to mold spores in the atmosphere, which are freely breathed, much like all-year-round pollen. These spores are only absent on cold, frosty days and when snow lies on the ground. At different times of the year, different fungi dominate.

There are some 4,000 indoor molds that flourish in our homes. Even an apparently dry house is subject to moisture from cooking, perspiration of the occupants and moisture exhaled in breathing.

Measurements show that an average family may give off up to 20 liters of moisture daily. Particularly bad areas for mold are rooms where the moisture is at its highest, such as the kitchen and bathroom. Of course, not all houses are structurally dry. Older property especially tends to be damp. Low-lying dwellings and those near rivers, lakes and marshes are also more damp than most.

Some homes are particularly bad for mold content and, indeed, it may be evident as green or black patches growing on the walls. Familiar 'dry rot' is a mold – Merulius lacrymans – despite its name, dry rot needs moisture to grow. Even when not visible, mold may be hidden in fabrics, carpets and furniture, especially if these are damp, old or have food particles embedded in them.

Mold In Our Diet

There is mold in our diet too. Not just in cheese and mushrooms, I am referring to unwanted molds. Bread is a shocking and surprising avenue of exposure.

In 1980 I found a survey that gave the following fungi in flour milled in the UK (dates from Food Surveillance Paper, HMSO, no 4, 1980):

- Penicillium,
- Cladosporium,
- Aspergillus candidus,
- Aspergillus flavus,
- Mucor,
- Aspergillus terreus,
- Alternaria,
- Aspergillus versicolor Absida,

- Aspergillus fumigatus,
- Verticullium and
- Paecilomyces

This diversity is typical for other countries.

Mold contamination of animal feeds can lead to further exposure. Both molds and toxins (along with antibiotics, hormones and sedatives) pass into dairy produce, meat, eggs, bacon and poultry.

As the molds' main port of entry is the mouth, the digestive tract tends to be the most affected. Darkness and moisture within the gut suit these organisms very well. Add to that the fact that our immune systems seem to be already under siege and, not surprisingly, we have a formula for trouble of epidemic proportions.

Malabsorption syndrome develops due to intestinal inflammation together with an inability to eliminate cellular waste. As my friend Dr Nancy Dunne in Dublin is inclined to put it, 'Pseudo-celiac disease with negative alpha-gliadin antibody titres and normal jejunal biopsy but full symptomatology of celiac disease is now as rife as the common cold.

And that was dear Nancy talking in the 1980s. It has only got worse!

It is possible, indeed probable, that many symptoms supposed to be mold allergy are actually the poisoning effects of traces of mycotoxins. Ergot mold contains a relative of LSD; 'magic mushrooms' contain a hallucinogen called psilocybin.

It isn't hard to imagine that there may be many more such chemical compounds, as yet undiscovered, lurking in molds.

I call the true mold allergic the 'moldy patient'. There seems to be a syndrome of reacting to dietary mold, damp weather, old musty buildings, etc.; the patient often has intestinal Candidiasis; cravings for sweets seem to be a major feature and tolerance of alcohol (yeast) is poor.

The Moldy Patient

Athlete's foot and skin infections with mold (ringworm or Tinea) may be present, suggesting the patient is somehow a breeding ground for molds.

For some reason I am unable to explain, but it is extremely common, mold-allergic patients become highly sensitive to ambient chemicals in the environment. Possibly molds are suppressing the enzymes of detoxification pathways in much the same way as they are capable of causing immune suppression.

Symptoms Suggesting Mold Sensitivity:

- Worse on damp days
- Worse in musty old buildings, with old fabrics and papers
- Cravings for sweet foods
- Cravings for bread and yeast foods
- Chemical hypersensitivity

- Poor tolerance of alcohol, craving for alcohol
- Skin infections with mold, e.g. troublesome athlete's foot
- Known Candidiasis
- Vaginal Thrush
- Fatigue
- Mood disorder, spacey 'unreal' feeling

I continue to use the concept of Candida or yeast in talking to patients since most people have heard of it and believe that is what they have got. However, I prefer the label I used in my Allergy Handbook (Thorsons, 1988), the so-called 'moldy patient'.

It is a term that stays in the mind, broadens out the debate and gives better insight into what we are dealing with. Whatever the nature of this illness, its manifestation is of a disease caused by encountering and being sensitized by biological products from yeasts, fungi and molds.

Patients are made worse by anything that can be fermented, such as starch and sugars; they react to foodstuffs containing yeast or mold (bread, wine, vinegar, etc.); they are often ill in moldy or musty surroundings (old buildings, woodlands or animal byres); some are even sensitive to damp weather, when molds are sporing freely; often there are accompanying infections of the fungus type including athlete's foot or other skin infections such as Tinea and Epidermophyton; finally, the patient may have been diagnosed as having Candida (Thrush), either in the mouth, gut or vagina.

Basically, this type of patient is a paradise for molds and yeasts, including Candida, to live in and on…

Testing Your Home For Mold

With the cooperation of a doctor or the local health laboratory, you can test your home for the presence of extensive molds. There are some in very home; it's simply a matter of quantity.

How it's done is by exposing laboratory plates coated with a growing medium to the general atmosphere in the home or you can limit this to a specific room. The plates are then covered, dashed off to the lab, where they culture whatever landed on the plates.

The longer the plates are left exposed, the more mold will gather, obviously.

A laboratory will be able to identify most mold species. Medical testing will tell you if you are sensitive to the common molds in your home.

You can get a home mold testing kit from here:

Home Mold Laboratory
3250 Old Farm Lane Ste 1
Walled Lake, MI 48390
1-877-665-3373
http://www.homemoldtestkits.com/

Getting Rid Of Molds

If mold is a problem, you need to get rid of it as much as possible.

The most important action to take is to eradicate damp where it exists. If these are structural problems to the building you must hire a qualified builder who can advise you what to do.

Rising damp, leaking gutters or faulty plumbing can all be fixed and need tacking definitively.

A dehumidifier may help dry out the indoor atmosphere. There are several models around now aimed at the domestic market, but be careful. Make sure that the moisture they collect doesn't become a focus for growth of mold and other pathogens.

Remove any obvious sources of mold contamination, such as old damp fabrics, lumber and other household waste. You may need to increase the efficiency of garbage disposal.

House plants, too, are sources of mold. Parting with them may be necessary in very severe cases. There are some very good artificial plants. If, like me, you love the sight of green foliage, even fakes are better than nothing.

Killing Mold And Spores

Once the problem is fixed, you can consider drastic reduction of the existing mold count in your home. The pros and cons need to be weighed: if someone in the house is very mold sensitive and there is a heavy presence of mold when tested, this should be a priority.

There are hazards to this procedure, so it should be undertaken with care.

We use formaldehyde, a gas which is toxic and kills mold and spores (one of the main reasons it is used as a preservative in the biology lab!) But it is also a danger to humans. It's not a "killer gas", such as hydrogen cyanide or phosgene. But long-term health effects of formaldehyde are bad and includes the possibility of cancer.

The procedure is simple enough: all doors and windows are closed and dishes or bowls of formaldehyde liquid are left uncovered in every room and passageway. It evaporates and fills the air with sterilizing fumes. It should be left to do its work as long as possible, preferably several days.

No-one is to linger in the house while this procedure is being done. This may mean taking a short vacation. Pets—and remember the goldfish, budgerigar or hamsters, or they will die—should be boarded out, if necessary.

Whoever is in charge of the procedure makes sure people and pets are safely outside the home. He or she then goes through room after room, pouring one or more dishes of formaldehyde (wide dished evaporate faster than bowls).

Leave the final room and hall passageway till last, of course. Then exit quickly (the fumes are very irritating to breathe) and lock the door.

On return, the procedure is reversed. The formaldehyde is removed and poured away (legally, whatever is required by law in your territory). Open all doors and windows and let fresh air circulate for several hours.

Only when the air is cleared and smell all but gone should occupancy be resumed.

Air Filtration

If you or someone in the family is very sensitive to molds and yeasts, it makes sense to filter the indoor air.

Many companies now produce personal environment air systems. These are a great boon to all who are allergic to environmental triggers, such as dust, pollen and animal danders: they ensure a clean local environment and they are very effective against airborne mold spores indoors.

Those which have HEPA filtration (high-efficiency particulate air) are by far the best. Same models will scrub the air of chemicals at the same time; a good idea and worth the extra investment.

Mycotoxins

Mycotoxins are a group of potent and often cancer-causing chemicals produced by a number of molds. This is not the same as allergy or infections with mold. This is poisoning.

LSD-related isoergine from the cereal mold ergot is an example. There is good reason to believe that the Salem witch "outbreak" was the result of mass hallucinations from ergot poisoning.

Most mycotoxins are present in insignificant quantities and many appear to pose no toxic threat to humans. But a few are deadly. Most people have heard of the potent liver poison and carcinogen aflatoxin B1, secreted by the common mold Aspergillus flavus that grows on wheat, maize, peanuts and other crops.

Many environmentalists regard aflatoxin B1 as the most powerful carcinogen known. Most mycotoxins survive cooking, so even this way of potentially neutralizing them is no good.

Nor is aflatoxin the only culprit. It appears there are plenty. Some species of Penicillium produce ochratosxin (on wet grains which may go on to contaminate offal meat). Ochratoxin-A can cause kidney damage.

A Fusarium toxin, deoxynibalenol (DON) has been linked indirectly to disorders of the immune system. DON is also known as vomitox in because it causes pigs that eat it to vomit. It may also be implicated in esophageal cancer.

Some mycotoxins have hormone activity. Zearalenone, another toxin from Fusarium, has been identified as a cause of abortion. Zearalenone and its derivatives mimic female sex hormones by binding to the same cellular receptors, as do estrogenic hormones. This gives rise to similar physiological and pathological effects.

The chief concern regarding human health is the possibility of such mycotoxins inducing hormone-dependent cancers such as cancer of the uterus. In addition to cancer, all these estrogen-like agents can produce fetal abnormalities.

CHAPTER 3

Dysbiosis and GMO

We now come to the bigger picture; a much bigger picture, that is.

For decades we've known that the problem with intestinal function is not really as simple as just Candida and yeasts. After decades of antibiotic use and abuse, we have reached a position where very few humans have natural healthy intestines. Instead they have lost much of their so-called "flora" and instead been invaded with troublesome, unhealthy microbes.

This might sound strange at first: aren't ALL microbes unhealthy?

The answer is, no, they are not. In our natural (I stress the word natural) and healthy state, our bodies are loaded with microorganisms that are crucial to our survival. They are needed to squeeze out unfriendly germs.

Some actually do good things for us, such as helping provide nutrients.

We call this disrupted healthy bowel flora "dysbiosis" (which means "wrong organisms", basically). Now it has emerged just in the last few years that we had no idea just how important, how damaging dysbiosis is and how widespread the effects of it spread beyond the intestines.

As a further complication, we now have to deal with GMO foods, including the deadly *Bacillus thuringiensis* (or Bt for short), which is supposed to be an insecticide but is tearing up the guts of humans and animals who encounter it.

The truth is the full picture is a lot bigger and more amazing (frankly), than I or my colleagues could ever have guessed in those early years. Dysbiosis is an exploding modern science with genetic and health implications for us all.Intelligent focus is now on a far bigger concept than just pathogens: I'm talking about the human microbiome.

The Human Microbiome

Let's start with an understanding of the good stuff, before we look at pathological changes.

The fact is, we live in a sea of bacteria. Not only that, but our bodies are inhabited by an on-board crowded colony of bacteria and other life forms, such as viruses, archea (like primitive bacteria), fungi, yeasts, protozoa and parasites.

Our bodies have been likened to a coral reef! Science writer Ed Young calls us "Humanville", a city where hundreds of trillions of denizens reside.

We are born free of organisms, thanks to the sterile conditions in the womb. But it doesn't last. Within hours, a multitude of microbes contacted during birth jump on board. In fact mother's gift at birth: the sweat, urine, vaginal secretions and fecal matter turns out to be absolutely vital to the child's healthy growth and development.

Without this "transplant" of germs the child would not grow up normally; it's immune system would not develop as it should; and even nervous system function would be severely compromised (fortunately, babies born by Caesararian get their "dose" from the surgical operatives and subsequent handling).

The Statistics

I already shared in my book "How To Survive In A World Without Antibiotics" that our dry body weight (minus all the water) is an amazing 10% bacteria and pathogens.

In fact, once grown, the average person is home to about 100 trillion microbes and they are everywhere, colonizing your gut, mouth, skin, mucous membranes and genitals.

The combined genetic content of this vast colony of organisms we have started to view as a whole and entire: we call it the microbiome (like the word "genome", but for microbes). What has been recently discovered is nothing short of STAGGERING: the bacterial genes in our gut can tell our bodies what to do, just as surely as our own genes!

What They Do For Us

They don't just sit there! These microbes interact with us *very beneficially*. A balanced and healthy gut flora helps keep disease-causing microbes at bay by occupying their preferred niches.

Premature babies who do not get their inoculation, since they are kept in strict hygienic conditions, are prone to a deadly bowel condition called necrotising enterocolitis. It kills up to 1 in 5 preemies. Doctors have failed to blame it on any one organism: in fact it seems that any abnormal combination of bacterial species in their stools could indicate which babies will get the disease.

But it's more than that even. Gut flora are also involved in the development of the immune system. The gut, being technically "outside" the body, is permanently in direct contact with the germ-infested outside world, contains a large amount of immune tissue (about 80% in Peyer's patches).

The immune system becomes educated by sampling the gut flora. In mice kept sterile of microbes, immune tissue fails to mature properly and carries fewer of the signaling molecules that sense and react to pathogens.

Microbes also help in the formation of gut structure. The tiny little "hairs" we use for absorption called villi depend on our normal population of microbes for their formation. Villi develop abnormally in microbe-free mice. Malabsorption—meaning poor nutrition because nutrients are not properly absorbed—is inevitable when this happens.

But perhaps most startling of all: our gut microbes help with valuable neurological development. We now understand something called the gut-brain axis. It was there all the time and even appears in our language: from "gut feelings" to "having some guts", English is full of phrases where our bowels exert an influence upon our behavior. There are open lines of communication between brains and bowels and, in animal tests at least, these channels allow an individual's gut bacteria to steer their behavior.

By studying mice, Rochellys Diaz Heijtz from the Karolinska Institute has found that a mammal's gut bacteria can affect the way its brain develops as it grows up. They could even influence how it behaves as an adult.

Under their influence, a baby's nerves will grow and connect in ways that will affect everything from how anxious to how coordinated it is. Thanks to that "messy" birth, an infant's brain is being shaped by its gut.

A New Organ

Our colony of microbial passengers is such a large entity and so influential on our health, it has been likened to an extra organ, like a liver, heart or lungs. It's the unseen force that processes much of Humanville's food supply, regulates its defences against invaders, and keeps it working like a healthy, well-oiled machine.

Our microbiome, it transpires, affects chronic diseases and the likelihood of obesity. They are essential to our digestion, by breaking down chemicals in our food that we wouldn't normally be able to process.

Each microbiome is very distinctive. It turns out that we can identify a species, or even an individual, form the genetic make up of these colonies. It's as individual as your passport or driving license!

A new study shows that the abundance of certain bacterial genes in your feces correlates with your age, sex, body mass index and nationality. Increasing age, for example, is associated with an increase in the genes for enzymes needed to break down starches in the diet. Men seem to have more biochemical pathways for the synthesis of the amino acid aspartate than women. The microbiomes of people with higher BMIs were richer in genes involved in harvesting energy from gut contents. And people from different countries had small subsets of genes associated with their nationality (Nature, DOI: 10.1038/nature09944).

No wonder then that blasting it all to hell with broad-spectrum antibiotics is a disaster. Health is about balance; once you upset the balance, total health is gone for good, unless you can somehow restore that balance.

Suddenly, dysbiosis (not a medially accepted term, by the way, but real nonetheless) start to look like a dangerous condition. We are in BIG trouble when this crowd gets displaced or goes out of sorts!

Metagenomics

Looking further at the vast collection of microbial DNA and genes we carry in our guts, it soon becomes obvious why all this is important.

For one thing, many species cannot be grown in the lab. The only way we have found them is because of their DNA imprint. You can't just swallow some, like it was *Acidophilus* or yoghurt!

All this is being extensively studied by Metagenomics of the Human Intestinal Tract (MetaHIT), a European Union-based consortium. The researchers studied fecal samples taken from 124

European adults and found a staggering 3.3 million different microbial genes, meaning that they outnumber our own human gene set about 150-fold (Nature, vol 464, p 59).

We are then, in effect, a sort of combined "super-organism" that functions as a whole which is more than just its parts.

So what do these microbiomic genes do? Many seem to be plugging metabolic gaps in our own genome. It is common knowledge that we are unable to synthesize enough vitamin B or any vitamin K without our gut flora, but microbes assume many other useful functions.

For example, they contain genes that convert complex carbohydrates into simpler molecules called short-chain fatty acids, an important energy source accounting for between 5 and 15 per cent of our requirements.

Other core genes break down plant cellulose and complex sugars such as pectin, found in fruit and vegetables, which allows us to digest foods we could not handle without them.

The MetaHIT project also found microbial genes that seem to be involved in metabolizing drugs and other non-dietary compounds, such as toxins and food additives.

So this is an entirely new twist on chemical sensitivity. It also fits entirely with my clinical observations, which I first published decades ago: that "Candida" or dysbiosis cases were usually extremely chemically sensitive (part of my "awesome foursome" syndrome, indicating dysbiosis).

So, "personalized" medicine just became vastly more complicated. This is an indirect inflammation, caused by a disordered microbiome.

When It Goes Wrong

So now we are beginning to get a much more technical and understandable view of what "dysbiosis" is really all about and why it is such a disaster.

A study published recently showed that gut flora composition alters dramatically in response to a course of antibiotics, before starting to rebuild itself after about a week (Proceedings of the National Academy of Sciences, vol 108, p 4554). "It does mostly bounce back but certainly not quite all the way," says Les Dethlefsen from Stanford University in California, one of the research team. He speculates that repeated disturbances of the ecological balance of the gut microbiome could permanently shift the functioning of the ecosystem - an alteration that would then be passed down from parent to child. "Every time we perturb the community, there is a roll of the dice," he says.

Among the participants in the MetaHIT project was a group of people with inflammatory bowel diseases such as ulcerative colitis and Crohn's disease. Previous research suggested that this group would have a lower diversity of bacterial species in their guts; that's a natural after-effect of frequent antibiotic use.

It follows, therefore, that they have fewer microbial genes. Sure enough, those in the MetaHIT study had 25 per cent less than healthy people.

Meanwhile, research in mice indicates that the balance of microbes in the gut can play a part in the development of type 2 diabetes. Gut flora might also be associated with obesity. When a team led by Jeffrey Gordon from Washington University in St Louis took microbes from the guts of lean and obese mice and transplanted them into germ-free mice, they found that those with the microbiome of obese mice put on significantly more weight (Nature, vol 444, p 1027). Subsequent studies indicate that the microbiomes of obese humans have a greater ability to harvest energy from food (Obesity, vol 18, p 190).

So you see that dysbiosis, as described here in full, is bound to result in ill health. It leads to a whole raft of conditions we are seeing today, such as diabetes, obesity, dementia and auto-immune disease. The old housewives' term "Candida" just doesn't cut it any more and should be dropped.

Bacillus Thuringiensis

Bacillus thuringiensis (Bt for short) is a naturally occurring microbe, found widely in the soil. It also occurs naturally in the gut of caterpillars of various types of moths and butterflies, as well on leaf surfaces, aquatic environments, animal feces, insect rich environments, flour mills and grain storage facilities

It has become infamous for its use in genetically modified organisms or GMO crops. Bt produces a toxin which inflames the guts of insects and bursts them open. So when pests feed on the crops, they are killed. But it does no harm whatever to humans… THEY CLAIM. Well, only a fool would believe that.

In fact Bt is a pernicious type of dysbiosis. It may even damage our own flora in the way that an antibiotic does. We just don't know! These products have been rushed to the market by irresponsible biotech corporations, such as Monsanto and Bayer CropScience and spread everywhere, without adequate safety testing.

B. thuringiensis-based insecticides are applied as liquid sprays on crop plants, where the insecticide must be ingested to be effective. Of course we humans too ingest the toxin, when we et the GM foods. Bt modified crops have been in your food supply since 1985, so if you can date your ill health from around that time, GMO foods may well be the cause.

We don't know yet what it does to human physiology, and that's the truth. But we do know, for sure, that people who give up eating genetically modified foods, recover their health; moreover distress of the bowel, typical of dysbiosis, clears up rapidly.

Biotech corporations such as Monsanto try to distort or deny the evidence, sometimes pointing to their own studies that supposedly show no reactions. But the longest test they conducted only lasted for 90 days. Would you accept the data that tobacco caused no harm after just 90 days of smoking?

Also, when scientists such as French toxicologist G.E. Seralini re-analyzed Monsanto's raw data, it actually showed that the rats fed GM corn suffered from clear signs of toxicity – evidence that industry scientists skillfully overlooked.

Doctors Are Starting To Prescribe Non-GMO Diets

Although there have been no human clinical trials, experts conclude that there is sufficient evidence from animal feeding studies to remove GMOs altogether. The American Academy of Environmental Medicine (AAEM) called for a moratorium in 2009 based on their review of the research. According to their former president, Dr. Robin Bernhoft, the Academy "recommends that all physicians should prescribe non-genetically modified food for all patients, and that we should educate all of our patients on the potential health dangers, and known health dangers of GMO food."

Today, thousands of physicians and nutritionists do just that, and they report that a wide variety of health conditions improve after people make the change. Here are some recent examples I culled from the work of internist Emily Lidner MD [http://vitalitymagazine.com/article/dramatic-health-recoveries-reported/ accessed 8.00 am BST 2/10/2010]:

1. Trial consultant LaDonna Carlton, had to take two pills, three times a day to suppress the painful cramps and constant diarrhea associated with her irritable bowel syndrome. "My doctor told me I would be on this forever," says LaDonna. But then she met Dr. Lindner. "The first thing she did," says LaDonna, "was take me off GMOs," including soy, corn, canola oil, and sugar. "Within two months," she says, "I didn't need the medication any longer."

    Since LaDonna stopped preparing foods with GMOs, her husband Fred was swept along with the new diet. And he's glad he was. "I feel 10 times better," he says. At 73, Fred plays full court basketball, even with two artificial knees. The new diet, he says, "made me feel much younger... I feel like I'm 50."

2. Interior designer, Carol Salb, also recovered from irritable bowel syndrome, as well as cold hands and feet, thinning hair, allergies, and daily congestion. "I felt better in two and half weeks [after going GMO-free]," she says. That was six years ago and she's still going strong.

3. We interviewed former school teacher Theresa Haerle on her 25th day on a GMO-free diet, and she had already shed more than 10 pounds. Even more remarkable was her recovery from 30 years of colitis – by the third day of her diet. In addition, her skin problems started to clear, she had more energy than she'd had in years, and it no longer hurt to get out of bed in the morning.

4. Kids are also recovering. One middle schooler changed his diet and no longer suffers from incapacitating migraines and asthma. Another recovered from horrible pain in his gut.

Dr. Lindner says, "I tell my patients to avoid genetically modified foods because in my experience, with those foods there is more allergies and asthma," as well as digestive issues such as gas, bloating, irritable bowel, colitis, and leaky gut.

"And what emanates from that," she says, "is everything. Lots of arthritis problems, autoimmune diseases, anxiety... neurological problems; anything that comes from an inspired immune system response."

The speed of recovery varies, usually depending on the symptom. "When I change people from a GMO diet to a GMO-free diet," she says, "I see results instantaneously in people who have foggy thinking and people who have gut symptoms like bloating, gas, irritation. In terms of allergies, it might take two to five days. In terms of depression, it starts to lift almost instantaneously. It takes from a day, to certainly within two weeks." Full results usually take about four to six weeks. Dr. Lindner doesn't just eliminate GMOs in her dietary regimen, but that, she says, is the most critical component.

You will readily see that patients with symptoms of supposed "Candida", leaky gut, bowel inflammation, IBS and many more health conditions should not eat GMO crops.

In fact none of us should. Appendix 2 will help you to avoid eating GMO foods.

CHAPTER 4

Candida Treatments & Research

There are really 5 basic approaches to eradicating Candida and yeasts:

1. Kill 'em
2. Starve 'em
3. Avoid foods of that class (yeasts, molds, cheese, etc.)
4. Squeeze 'em Out. Set up competitive friendly microbes (probiotics)
5. Clean up the terrain

One, two or three actions is better than none but it is possible to do all five.

Kill 'Em: Anti-microbials

To destroy micro-organisms is a familiar concept to most doctors. They think in terms of antibiotics, anti-fungals, anti-parasites drugs and similar medications.

True enough, anti-fungals are a critical part of the armoury against Candida and yeasts. Nystatin, ketoconazole and amphotericin B are medicines in this class.

But it is also possible to use more natural, "holistic" substances to achieve the same effect. Mountain savory, for example, has scientifically-proven properties against fungus and mold. So has garlic. These are not as powerful but then, they are not as risky either!

I'll return to the use of anti-fungals in a later section.

Starve 'Em: Diet Changes

If you are trying to eradicate a hostile organism, it doesn't make sense to go on supplying its favorite foods! All fermenting organisms, of which yeast and Candida are examples, like to turn sugars into alcohol, releasing food energy in the process. We call this fermentation.

We rely in fermentation to make our boozy beverages, such as beer and wine. Yeast will take the sugar in grapes and turn it into alcohol, producing wine in the process (very tasty wine, if you do it right).

While battling Candida, therefore, and especially in the early stages of the cure process, you must strictly avoid all sugar substances. This means more than just granulated white sugar that you put in tea and coffee. It means all hidden sugar in your diet.

Food manufacturers love to sneak sugar into their foodstuffs. Their logic is that if it tastes nice (sweet) people will want more and probably get hooked on it. Thus they make more sales. Sugar is added to ludicrous things today, like French fries, humus, bread and toothpaste (rot your teeth while cleaning them!)

So as well as avoiding added sugar, you need to avoid all manufactured foods. Eat only fresh whole foods.

Avoid fruit juices, which are often sweetened with extra sugar. Even those which are not still have too high a sugar content. What's more fruit juice contains a lot of mold. You want to avoid mold contacts as much as possible.

Some writers foolishly recommend avoidance of fruit and similar natural foods. This may lead to dangerous inadequacies in nutrition and is bad advice because it isn't necessary. Anyone with 'Candida' made ill by eating fruit has a fruit allergy, almost certainly.

Those who feel unwell after eating sugars may really have a degree of carbohydrate intolerance due to deficient enzymes (not so rare) and it is NOT, as some imaginative women insist, their "Candida" getting free in the blood.

Best advice: just go easy and avoid the very sugary fruits, such as banana, dates and figs. Most berries are low in sugar. Be guided by the glycemic index: the higher the index, the more available sugar.

Avoid all starches for the same reason. Refined flour translates into quite a lot of sugar or equivalent. Pasta, pastries, muffins and pancakes are all bad news EVEN BEFORE ANY SUGAR OR SWEETENING IS ADDED.

Here are some examples of the glycemic index of foods:

Muesli	43
Oat bran	55
Quick oats	66
Corn flakes	92
Dates	100
Banana	60 - 70
Strawberries	40
Grapefruit	25
Cherries	22

Honey, agave and maple syrup are also banned. These are very sugar-rich. Don't fall for the propaganda on agave nectar: it's mainly added sugar.

Don't ever believe a manufacturer's label which says "sugar free". It will probably have HFCS (high fructose corn syrup) or some similar fraud.

Sugar-Substitutes
What about stevia, aspartame, Splenda and other substitutes? This is a common and obvious question.

I definitely don't recommend these as a solution. They are extremely sweet; hundreds of times sweeter than sugar. This gives your palate the wrong signals. You want LESS sweetness in your life not more!

Just avoid any alternative sweeteners and get used to it. After a couple of weeks off sugar you'll find even a carrot tastes sweet; there's quite a lot of sugar in a carrot. You'll be amazed to find that when you go back to tea or coffee with sugar, it will taste disgustingly sweet!

Avoiding yeasts, molds and ferments in food
You need to avoid what are similar foodstuffs to yeast. It's just adding to the body's total burden of ferments and that's what has been making you sick.

There is a whole class of living organisms which are similar in nature: they are good at breaking down organic substances, digesting them and removing them from the environment.

Mold is a classic example. Mold will eliminate dead plants and animals by digesting the bodies. This property of mold is a nuisance when it comes to our food: moldy food is contaminated and cannot be eaten. But if mold didn't do this, we would be neck deep in corpses everywhere on planet Earth!

Molds re-cycle us!

In reality, we take advantage of this class of foods in other ways. Cheese, for example, is made by mold. The blue cheeses are especially rich in it; the blue "veins" are in fact blue-green mold, like penicillin.

There is more about foods to avoid later and what substitutes to use. Also, the appendix gives a list of foods that contain, or may contain, yeasts and ferments.

Sqeeze 'Em Out: The Use Of Probiotics

I explained earlier that most fungal and yeast overgrowth in our bodies comes from the indiscriminate use of antibiotics. This wipes out friendly microbes, which live in us and on us (we need them). As a result, hostile organisms are given a strong advantage and may multiply rapidly to fill the spaces left by the organisms which were wiped out.

Think of it in gardening terms. If you have a healthy garden, filled with flourishing healthy plants, it is very difficult for weeds to get a hold. But if you clear a bed of all useful flowers and leave it empty, weeds will overgrow it in no time. And, as every gardeners knows, once the weeds get a grip it is very, very difficult to dislodge them. Good plants won't flourish. You may need to weedkiller the lot and start again. It can be a heartbreaking disaster.

But our bodies are more resilient than a garden. If we set the conditions right, we can encourage the growth of friendly bacteria and other organisms, which then squeeze out the intruders. In gardening terms, it's like clearing a patch and planting good vigorous flowers, which then lock out the weeds from that particular spot.

As you keep going, gradually there are more and more good plants and fewer and fewer weeds.

The good flowers we introduce are called "probiotics". These are chosen carefully to be suitable for our bodies and to have the capability of beating out something vicious, like Candida or Gardia.

The most popular, traditionally, has been yoghourt. This is an idea that was started around 1910 by a man called Elie Metchnikoff (1845- 1916). Today we are less impressed by his evidence but there was a germ of an idea (no pun!)

Since then we have gone onto whole groups of probiotics, including Lactobacillus acidophilus from yoghurt (but not cow's yoghurt, as I will explain).

What is exciting is that now conventional medicine has begun to wake up to the probiotics idea and literally thousands of scientific studies are carried out and published each year on this topic. It's no longer "alternative" medicine (but it is still holistic).

44

Learn Your Probiotics

It makes sense to try and re-colonize the bowel with friendly bacteria. Most well known among these friendly bacteria is Lactobacillus acidophilus, the yoghourt-making germ.

Many supplements of 'acidophilus' are currently being marketed. Some contain very few live bacteria, if any, and are of poor value if not completely fraudulent.

In fact Bifidobacteria is much more prevalent in the gut, comprising some 90 per cent of natural bowel flora. Top brand probiotics, as these flora supplements are known, now include primarily Bifidobacteria. It makes sense.

Here's another caution: look for those that provide human-strain acidophilus; logically these are more likely to establish themselves in the human colon.

The Best Probiotics?

The product I used to recommend most was Probion® by the Swedish firm Wasa Medicals. Its strength is a special manufacturing process in which the tablets are pressed very lightly, so not crushing the living organisms.

Nowadays the best choices would be Lactobacillus rhamnosus, as lcr35, from Lyocentre, in Aurillac, France [Laboratoires Lyocentre, 24, avenue Georges Pompidou, Z.I. de Sistrières - BP 429, 15004 AURILLAC Cedex France)] and Bifidobacterium animalis subspecies lactis (BB12) from Chr. Hansen, Denmark [Chr. Hansen, Bøge Allé 10-12, DK-2970 Hørsholm, Denmark].

LCR35

One study of lcr35 investigated women with Nugent scores between 7 and 10 by vaginal swab (a measure of vaginal infestation). All women were treated with standard antibiotic therapy for 7 days. Women in the intervention group received vaginal capsules containing live Lcr35 for 7 days after antibiotic treatment; controls received none. Final vaginal swabs for Nugent scoring were taken 4 weeks after the last administration of the study medication. A highly significant number of women in the intervention group showed a drop the Nugent score of at least 5 grades, compared to fewer in the control group.

BB12

A study in a group of young adult women in south India showed that BB12 probiotic yoghurt was well tolerated and that fecal excretion of secretory immunoglobulin A was significantly increased during feeding of probiotic yoghurt compared to the baseline. Although the levels decreased after probiotic yoghurt was stopped, they did not return to normal and tended to be higher than baseline levels. This suggests that the effect of the probiotic yoghurt persisted even after cessation of feeding this.

[Nutrition Journal 2011, 10:138 doi:10.1186/1475-2891-10-138].

See Hansen's customer sheet here: http://cdn.chr-hansen.com/fileadmin/user_upload/ dokumenter/Probiotics_for_Human_Health/Product_Offerings_with_product_examples.pdf

Pre-Biotics

That may be a new term to you. Interestingly, it's even moved into orthodox medical thinking, where probiotics are now a hot topic of interest. Lots of scientific studies are emerging, making the value of pre- and probiotics very clear.

That's very different to when I was prescribing them over 20 years ago, when it was considered little better than snake oil!

What we mean by pre-biotics is food and support for the probiotics organisms.

These are, essentially, non-digestible food ingredients that stimulate the growth and/or activity of bacteria in the digestive system which are beneficial to the health of the body. They were first identified and named by Marcel Roberfroid in 1995. They are considered a functional food.

Typically, pre-biotics are carbohydrates (such as oligosaccharides), but the definition does not preclude non-carbohydrates. The common ones are nutritionally classed as soluble fiber. To some extent, many forms of dietary fiber exhibit some level of prebiotic effect.

Traditional dietary sources of prebiotics include soybeans, inulin sources (such as Jerusalem artichoke*, jicama, and chicory root), raw oats, unrefined wheat, unrefined barley and yacon. The great thing is that pre-biotics (and probiotics to an extent) have been shown to boost the immune system directly. That's just what we want when we are trying to eradicate a difficult infectious organism.

Some of the oligosaccharides that naturally occur in breast milk are believed to play an important role in the development of a healthy immune system in infants.

*Jerusalem artichoke is the star pre-biotic, because of the amount of fiber it holds (over 30%).

Unsightly Nail Fungus

One of the troublesome conditions to plague "moldy patients" is that of nail fungus or Onychomycosis. This mainly affects the toes, causing them to turn yellow, soften, swell and distort, so the foot looks quite ugly and embarrassing.

There are lots of supposed remedies, some marketed quite fraudulently in my opinion.

Podiatrists (chiropodists to the British) recommend iso-propyl alcohol (no, don't write and tell me Hulda Reger Clark's crackpot theories, thank you).

Tea Tree oil I think is a better bet. But how about this for a good idea: deliberately infecting your nails with another (safe) fungus which literally EATS the nail fungus. It then dies and disappears.

This "cannibal fungus" is called Pythium oligandrum and is a totally safe, 100% natural treatment (external use) against harmful skin/nail fungi. This mycoparasite eats the "Tinea" dermatophyte fungi that cause Athlete's foot, nail fungus (Onychomycosis), jock itch and ringworm. When the bad fungi are all gone, the Pythium disappears too.

And yes, there is science: human studies in fact:
http://pythium-oligandrum.owndoc.com/pythium-oligandrum-study.html

You can learn more about this and get some supplies by starting with this book: http://pythium-oligandrum.owndoc.com/pythium-oligandrum.pdf

Fungal Sinusitis

You may be one of the unlucky people troubled by fungal sinusitis. This can be caused by Candida albicans or any one of a number of molds/funguses. What can you do to clear it?

First: you MUST get rid of the mold, fungus, whatever, from your environment. If you just keep breathing it in again, you are wasting time and money on treatment. If the source of mold is in your workplace, you must take it up with the company doctor or health officer.

It makes most sense to work with a health professional and get a fungal culture from an intranasal swab. You may also be able to arrange to have culture plates set around your home, to see what's growing there and compare it to the infectious species. This is basic detective work.

Fungal sinusitis will generally surrender to one of the following treatments:

- Quinton nasal spray (favorite)
- Hydrogen peroxide protocol alternating with EDTA
- Ozone ear insufflation (actually, ozone anywhere will work)
- Neil Med washes (Neti pots)
- Compounded antifungal nasal sprays (Lee Silsby in Ohio compounds flucanizole, Itraconizole and ketoconizole nasal sprays).

Clean Up The Terrain. The Answer To Chronic Candida.

One thing I learned for sure over the decades of treating this condition: if you don't fix the thing that led to Candida/yeast overgrowth in the first place, then it will just come back. This is only logical!

Persistent problems with recurring Candida or yeasts were an absolute giveaway to other health problems. In that sense then, it was helpful, pointing to ways to improve overall health.

Providing that patients followed advice, took their anti-fungals, kept away from sugar and ferments, then if the condition still wouldn't clear—or just came back after a few weeks—I knew for certain there was heavy metal poisoning.

We call this sort of health issue one of "terrain". It has to do with the soil and seed metaphor. If you scatter seeds on the ground, if it is very infertile hostile soil, the seeds won't grow and flourish. They need water and nutrients.

So if the seed grows easily, you know that growing conditions are just perfect. If Candida grows and flourishes, you know your body is a sporting ground for pathogens.

We don't want that.

What it means is that the body's own defences, notably the immune and reticulo-endothelial systems, are not functioning properly. Something is turning off the natural healthy immune response.

Part of this is due to toxins released by the Candida itself. But time and again I came back to the fact that chronic Candida was a sign of weak terrain. Heavy metals are notorious for this effect, being among the most toxic substances we put into our environment. I'm talking now about lead, mercury, cadmium, aluminium, beryllium, arsenic and hexa-valent chromium.

Incidentally, some of these metals are known to cause cancer, presumably also because they block the normal workings of the immune system (the movie "Erin Brockovich" with Julia Roberts, was about hexa-valent chromium escaping into the environment).

If you have chronic or recurring Candida, you MUST give attention to the matter of heavy metal poisoning. Getting rid of these metals is a process of de-tox; one that we call "chelation" (from the Greek chela, or claw, meaning to snatch something away).

For years, alternative doctors have chelated out heavy toxic metals, using the IV approach. This is not suitable for home use or Candida therapy. Does oral chelation work effectively?

Well, if you listen to my friend Garry Gordon (www.gordonresearch.com) you'll think it does. He has accumulated over 500 papers on his website, showing scientifically that oral chelation is highly beneficial.

His recommendation includes oral EDTA and zeolite. I'm not impressed by the science on zeolite (much of it is invented and fraudulent). But Dr. Gordon is a committed fan. You choose.

There is no question about the EDTA. It works. Avoid the ridiculously priced suppository preparations. These are a rip of: there is no evidence that rectal EDTA has any benefits and, since this stuff is cheaper than aspirin, the price makes it a rip off.

EDTA is quite safe and is added to many food preparations.

Other chelation substances

Still not sure? Like all natural?

Well, remember toxic heavy metals are not supposed to be in our environment, so there is no "natural" chelator, really.

But apple pectin helps; so does garlic (surprisingly) and kelp.

But chlorella definitely warrants a mention. It's known as the natural "metal magnet". Numerous research projects in the U.S. and Europe indicate that chlorella can aids the body in breaking down persistent pesticides and metallic toxins such as mercury, cadmium and lead, DDT and PCB while strengthening the immune system response. In Japan, interest in chlorella has focused largely on its detoxifying properties - its ability to remove or neutralize poisonous substances from the body.

This detoxification of heavy metals and other chemical toxins in the blood will take 3 to 6 months to build up enough to begin this process depending on how much chlorella a person is taking.

It is a fibrous material which greatly augments healthy digestion and overall digestive track health, acting as a pre-biotic. It undoubtedly "mops up" metals, so binding them in its fiber net, as well as any other properties.

Chlorella is also thought to boost the immune system and help fight infection. It has been shown to increase the good bacteria in the gastrointestinal (GI) tract, which helps to treat Candida and other bowel infections. In other words, it is a mild probiotics in its own right.

Finally, chlorella provides all of the dietary-essential amino acids in excellent ratios. It is also a reliable source of essential fatty acids that are required for many important biochemical functions, including hormone balance. Chlorella also contains high levels of chlorophyll, beta-carotene and RNA/DNA. More than 20 vitamins and minerals are found in chlorella, including iron, calcium, potassium, magnesium, phosphorous, pro-vitamin A, vitamins C, B1, B2, B2, B5, B6, B12, E and K, biotin, inositol, folic acid, plus vitamins C, E and K.

Usual dose: 2- 6 X 500 mgm tablets daily.

Warning: (gotta say this!) Chlorella supplements can be rich in vitamin K, which can reduce the effectiveness of the blood-thinning drug Warfarin. Check with your physician if you are on any kind of anticoagulant.

Also chlorella increases uric acid levels and may be unsuitable for anyone with gout (gout is a rheumatic disease resulting from deposition of uric acid crystals (monosodium urate) in tissues and fluids within the body).

Finally, of course, you will want to avoid the contraceptive pill. That's a good idea anyway. According to current thinking the dramatic drop in the incidence of breast cancer was caused by the fact that more and more women were refusing to take "The Pill".

Conventional Medications For Yeast Infection

The rest of this chapter is going to focus on the anti-Candida drug medications that you can buy over the counter or get from your doctor to treat Candida.

There are some anti-fungal treatments that can actually kill the yeast. However, the problem with that is three fold:

Firstly, it may be a temporary fix only. Because yeast infection is a very complex condition, in order to expel the condition you need to neutralize the conditions that cause it to overgrow. As such, unless you get to the root of the problem it will grow again (much like a plant if you cut the leaves off)

Secondly, Candida is a pleomorphic organism. This means it changes form and will develop resistance to anti-fungal treatments.

Thirdly, most anti-fungal treatments have side effects. Some of these can be serious which means they can only be used for a short time.

Over the counter medicines

Generally over the counter medicines are aimed only at treating an infection in one particular area of the body. Creams, ointments and lotions are of this type. The purpose is to contain the condition in that area and prevent it from spreading.

For women, there are creams that you can buy over the counter, such as Canesten (Clotrimazole). These creams are applied to the vagina area, with an applicator.

For men, the cream needs to be applied to the penis area.

Gynazole is another very potent yeast infection cream. It is applied to the vagina or the penis area when the yeast infection is located. The active ingredient in Gynazole is called Butoconazole.

Women also have the option of using suppositories that are placed in the vagina and left to dissolve with body heat. This will release the active ingredients into the infected area.

For athlete's foot and jock itch, Miconazole ointment may work better or Ketoconazole (Daktarin). Daktacort is a proprietary formulation which also includes hydrocortisone, to reduce the itching and inflammation.

You can also find topical creams that can be bought over the counter. These are used to deal with the uncomfortable symptoms of Candida. These things include itching, burning and inflammation.

Over the counter medications are readily available without a prescription, and are also very inexpensive. They are also easy to use and fast acting in relieving the symptoms. However the disadvantages of using yeast infection creams and suppositories are:

• Over the counter medications can have serious side effects for pregnant women and those girls under the age of twelve.

• They only work temporality and alleviate the symptoms. They don't get to the root cause of the problems of yeast or Candida infection. Also, while you are using them, you may inadvertently create resistance to the medication.

• They are unable to provide a solution for more widespread Candida/yeast infection. This is because the medication can only be used locally in the affected areas. Systemic Candida is a problem that affects other areas of the body besides those where the symptoms are present (and where the condition began).

• The medications can be very messy to apply. They are also known to break down the material of birth control methods such as condoms.

Yeast Infection Prescription Medication

If you have tried over the counter treatment but have not responded well, your doctor may prescribe a medication for you. These will be more powerful and are usually taken orally, in the form of a pill.

As I wrote in the previous chapter, your doctor will take a swab and send it to the lab. Following the results, the doctor will offer you medication based on the severity of the yeast infection, and depending on whether you have other types of yeast infection.

Drugs are not the full solution. While they can be dramatically effective, taking meds does NOT solve the problem of why you got Candida in the first place!

If your diet is bad, you have poor teeth (for example) and so continue taking antibiotics or your immune system is compromised I any way, then the problem will simply recur.

Recurring or chronic Candida/yeast is usually a symptom of what I call the terrain: meaning, the tissues of your body are not healthy and favor the growth of something like yeasts or even bacteria.

Heavy metal toxicity is the usual reason for this and chronic or difficult Candida is a give-away sign of mercury, lead or other metal poisoning.

The Heavy Artillery

We now come to the powerful range of drugs which can quickly deal with an outbreak of yeast of Candida. Unqualified holistic practitioners are not licensed to prescribe these drugs, which is why you will often hear them claim they are no good anyway (sour grapes!)

I've been treating Candida and yeast overgrowth for over a quarter of a century; trust me: this is the quick and effective way.

But you do have to take care of all the other steps of my anti-mold/anti-yeast program:

A successful anti-mold and yeast killing program must include effective restoration of bowel flora.

The most important step is medication with suitable anti-fungal drugs. These must be prescribed by a competent physician.

Many of the modern anti-fungal drugs, but by no means all, belong to the azole class. These are indeed the heavy artillery and potentially toxic. Most place a burden on the liver and liver function tests should be carried out by your physician on a regular basis: not less than every 3 months (meaning at least every 3 months).

It may be a good idea to take sylymarin (milk thistle):

Silymarin

Silymarin is known to protect the liver. It's been used for liver support since ancient Roman times (when they used to drink till incapacitated and then take milk thistle to undo the effects of the carousing). It stimulates the manufacture of new liver cells, and increases the production of glutathione and bile.

But there is a bonus to silymarin. I came across a paper showing it has been found particularly useful in long-standing cases of chronic Candidiasis. Candida Albicans essentially can choke the liver, causing a domino effect of adverse events. Thus, by strengthening the liver, you enhance the attack against the yeast overgrowth. [Scand. J Gastroenterology, 1982; 17: 417-21; Min Med 1985; 72:26-79-88; J. Hepatol, 1989; 9: 105-13].

Safety

All these are powerful substances with potential toxicity. They need handling with skill. Repeated liver function tests may be necessary. It has to be said that these drugs are not suitable for every case.

They should NEVER be taken without consulting a physician. Do not be tempted to use tablets or capsules from a friend's prescription "to see if they work".

If these warnings worries you, let me tell you that over a space of 25 years I prescribed them regularly and never had one patient who got into trouble. It only requires care and common sense on the part of the practitioner to avoid complications.

If you want to limit yourself to alternative remedies, you may have a tougher battle but there is no reason you cannot win in the end (providing you take care of the diet and terrain issues I shall be talking about later.

First, let's start with an old favorite of mine and many pioneer physicians of the 80s and 90s.

Nystatin

Nystatin is the most popular anti-fungal drug. Even among people with allergies, it is well tolerated. The usual doses are in the range of 1,000,000 units, which is equal to a quarter of a teaspoon.

It comes as tablets, oral suspension, lozenges (pastilles), vaginal pessaries and cream.

But we pioneers found it had by far the best effect on generalized Candida when taken as the powder. It is virtually insoluble and goes through the bowel, like a scouring powder! For that reason taking the powder is a very non-toxic mode of administration.

As I said, it is well tolerated. The main side effects (not usually seen with the powder preparation) are nausea (sometimes vomiting), diarrhea (when taken orally), and local rashes and irritation.

The starting dose for the powder is a quarter of a teaspoon, four times a day.

Remember: Nystatin can act as a chelating agent (that is, it binds to metals and blocks them) and so should not be taken with nutritional supplements (it would remove zinc, magnesium etc.).

Nystatin is an antibiotic which is both fungistatic and fungicidal in vitro against a wide variety of yeasts and yeast-like fungi, including Candida albicans, C. parapsilosis, C. tropicalis, C. guilliermondi, C. pseudotropicalis, C. krusei, Torulopsis glabrata, Tricophyton rubrum, T. mentagrophytes.

Nystatin acts by binding to sterols in the cell membrane of susceptible species resulting in a change in membrane permeability and the subsequent leakage of intracellular components. On repeated subculturing with increasing levels of nystatin, Candida albicans does not develop resistance to Nystatin.

Generally, resistance to nystatin does not develop during therapy. However, other species of Candida (C. tropicalis, C. guilliermondi, C. krusei, and C. stellatoides) become quite resistant on treatment with nystatin and simultaneously become cross resistant to amphotericin as well. This resistance is lost when the antibiotic is removed.

Nystatin exhibits no appreciable activity against bacteria, protozoa, or viruses.

[Nystatin, by the way, stands for New York State Institute of Health]

Polyene Anti-fungals

Nystatin belongs to a class of anti-fungal drugs called the polyenes. Others include Rimocidin, Natamycin, Filipin and Candicin.

Amphotericin B (Fungilin, Fungizone, Abelcet, AmBisome, Fungisome, Amphocil, Amphotec) is one of the best known polyene alternatives to Nystatin.

In cases of severe systemic Candida (a kind of septicemia) it may be required intravenously, to save a person's life. But putting it directly into the blood is very dangerous. This would only happen under hospital care, so don't even think about it.

Amphotericin B, has finally been licensed as an oral liquid in the United States, and can be legally compounded by pharmacies in the U.S. It has been prescribed in this form for decades in Europe and elsewhere. Used in this way it is virtually non-toxic.

Liposomal complexes may be the best way to take Amphotericin B, to beat any side effects. Fungisome, Amphotec and Abelcet are liposomal preparations of Amphotericin B.

[Amphotericin A, if you are curious, doesn't work!]

The Azole Drugs

The remaining important anti-fungals are known as the azole group (imidazoles, triazoles and thiazoles). They work by inhibiting the fungus' ability to create cell walls. We don't need to bog down in the technicalities of this classification.

The main drugs you will encounter are as follows:

Fluconazole (Diflucan)

Until the advent of generics, this used to be very expensive. It is still costly. Comes in 75 mgm capsules, one a day for a week to ten days. A 'one-shot' form exists (150 mgm), for those likely to develop reactions to medication. Lengthy treatments should not be undertaken, as side effects are potentially serious.

Diflucan is a very potent pill that works as an anti-fungal. It was created to kill the Candida yeast and all types of fungus that have taken hold in your body. As I said, there are side effects and it should only be taken one time. Do not use this if you are pregnant.

Nizoral (Ketoconazole)

Nizoral is a stronger pill than Diflucan. It is also taken orally and is usually prescribed with other antibiotics in a combination. The aim of this medication is to kill Candida and other fungal forms.

This is another drug that is very easy to use, but it has potentially serious side effects. It can damage the liver. Before starting to take Nizoral, and at frequent intervals while you are taking it, you should have blood tests to evaluate your liver function.

Tell your doctor immediately if you experience any signs or symptoms that could mean liver damage: these include unusual fatigue, loss of appetite, nausea or vomiting, jaundice, dark urine, or pale stools.

Possible food and drug interactions when taking Nizoral

If Nizoral is taken with certain other drugs, the effects of either could be increased, decreased, or altered. It is especially important to check with your doctor before combining Nizoral with the following:

   Alcoholic beverages
- Antacids such as Di-Gel, Maalox, Mylanta, and others
- Anticoagulants such as Coumadin, Dicumarol, and others
- Anti-ulcer medications such as Axid, Pepcid, Tagamet, and Zantac
- Astemizole (Hismanal)
- Cisapride (Propulsid)
- Cyclosporine (Sandimmune, Neoral)
- Digoxin (Lanoxin)
- Drugs that relieve spasms, such as Donnatal
- Isoniazid (Nydrazid)
- Methylprednisolone (Medrol)
- Midazolam (Versed)
- Oral diabetes drugs such as Diabinese and Micronase
- Phenytoin (Dilantin)
- Rifampin (Rifadin, Rifamate, and Rimactane)
- Tacrolimus (Prograf)
- Terfenadine (Seldane)
- Theophyllines (Slo-Phyllin, Theo-Dur, others)
- Triazolam (Halcion)
- Nizoral comes in 200 mgm tablets.

Do NOT take Nizoral if you are pregnant or breast-feeding, even if your doctor assures you it is OK (and change your doctor immediately!)

Sporanox (Itraconazole)

Itraconazole must not be used with certain heart medications because very serious, possibly fatal reactions may occur, such as irregular heartbeats (arrhythmias). Itraconazole blocks the breakdown of these medications by the liver causing buildup of these drugs in your body.

Itraconazole should not be used to treat fungal nail infections if you have heart disease (congestive heart failure), because it may worsen congestive heart failure. Seek immediate medical attention if you develop swelling of the feet/ankles, sudden weight gain, or trouble breathing.

Sporanox comes in 100 mgm tablets. Dosing regimes vary but it may be a good idea to take it one week on and three weeks off (1 week per month).

Others (For Completeness)

Benzoic acid – has antifugal properties but must be combined with a keratolytic agent such as in Whitfield's Ointment.

- Ciclopirox – (ciclopirox olamine), most useful against Tinea versicolour (vitiligo)
- Tolnaftate – marketed as Tinactin, Desenex, Aftate, or other names
- Undecylenic acid – an unsaturated fatty acid derived from natural castor oil;
- fungistatic as well as anti-bacterial and anti-viral
- Flucytosine or 5-fluorocytosine – an antimetabolite

Griseofulvin – binds to polymerized microtubules and inhibits fungal mitosis. You may be offered this for bad toenails and fingernails (onychomycosis). It is a notorious liver toxin and you should not take it if you have ever had hepatitis, glandular fever or a history of heavy drinking. I took it when I was in my twenties, for athlete's foot. It was a near disaster: I went jaundiced within a few days and would now probably die if I tried it again. You become super-sensitized.

Haloprogin. You may also come across written accounts of this drug – it has been discontinued due to the emergence of safer anti-fungals, with fewer side effects

> Your doctor may want to prescribe you an anti- depressant, like amitryptiline. This is supposed to be a sedative that has a mild analgesic (painkilling) effect which can help relieve pain at night. Don't take it! You're not depressed! You have a problem. I can show you how to fix it. Most doctors can't. But don't let them cover up their failure by implying half the problem is in your head!

A word about "die off" and so-called Herxeimer's

Much is disseminated about the 'burn off' or "die off" reaction patients sometime get when first starting anti-fungal treatment.

Candida die off, sometimes referred to as the Herxheimer Reaction, occurs when the excess Candida yeasts in our system literally "die off", producing toxins at too rapid a rate for the body to process and eliminate (named after Karl Herxeimer, who first described this reaction when syphilis was treated successfully, and is seen in 50% of patients with primary syphilis and about 90% of patients with secondary syphilis; it was caused by a flood of circulating dead spirochetes).

Burn-off (a sudden exacerbation of symptoms) does exist but is much exaggerated and rarely amounts to anything serious. Discontinuance allows it to settle and, nine times out of ten, when the patient resumes the treatment there is no further trouble.

In a sense it is a good, meaning you have slaughtered some of the enemy, but it can seem quite scary. Patients may rebel and try to stop therapy, thinking "It isn't working" or "The treatment is making me sick", when in fact it means the treatment is doing good.

As the body works to detoxify, you may experience symptoms including dizziness, headache, "foggy" headedness, fatigue, general malaise, depression, anxiety, heightened anger reactions, gas & bloating, flatulence, diarrhea, constipation, joint pain, muscle pain, body aches, sore throat, sweating, chills, nausea, skin breakouts, or other symptoms.

Doesn't sound good, does it? But try to be patient. Or stop the treatment for a few days and then resume. As I said, most often there is no problem on resuming.

Natural Anti-Fungal Treatments

There are many alternative solutions to the Candida problem. Most you can buy over the counter. Some you need to go to specialist suppliers. It's tempting to say search the Internet but I know you will find a lot of loopy advice out there, from people who want your money more than they want your recovery in health. Just take care!

These natural remedies are much more suitable for the self-help arena. Just don't expect results quite so fast (and don't expect ANY RESULTS AT ALL, if you don't do the other things I've been telling you in this book, such as diet changes).

What you have just read about "die off" may also apply to gentler holistic remedies. So be warned.

Garlic Definitely Helps

We all know garlic has surprising anti-fungal and antibiotic properties. What few people realize, however, is that most garlic preparations sold online and in health stores are worthless.

The anti-microbial activity comes from a compound called allicin. That's the stinky part of garlic, which is formed only when the clove is bruised or crushed. It's plentiful in fresh garlic.

There's none in garlic oil and capsules.

I would say to you save your money and go get fresh cloves from the supermarket. Crush them and eat them, add them to juice in the blender, and learn to live with the smell!

Garlic oil contains little allicin, due to the heat extraction process: thus a great deal of the antimicrobial function is lost. It is possible to get cold-pressed sources but be sure suppliers are being honest with you (there are a lot of liars selling health supplements on the Internet).

But you could try Kyolic (aged garlic). My friend Garry Gordon swears by it. I don't believe it has any value as an anti-microbial. I'm telling you this, in case I'm wrong!

Louis Pasteur commented on the bactericidal (bacteria – killing) effect of fresh garlic juice when dropped onto growing bacterial colonies. Over the years studies have shown that fresh garlic juice inhibits the growth of Staphylococcus (wound infection), Brucella, Salmonella (Typhoid) and several other bacteria. Indeed, its action was comparable in the laboratory with that of several antibiotics including penicillin, streptomycin, chloramphenicol, tetracycline and erythromycin.

But the action of garlic on yeast and fungi is perhaps even more dramatic. One study showed that growth of all soil fungi was totally inhibited by an aqueous garlic extract. Medically-important fungi and yeasts (notably Candida albicans are also inhibited and then killed by increasing concentrations.

Garlic, of course, has no real side-effects, other than stinky breath! It can be used indefinitely in quite large amounts (the patient's nearest and dearest permitting!)

Capricin

Capricin, a trade brand of caprylic acid, has been frequently advocated as an anti-fungal. It's a naturally occurring compound in our bodies and adding to its presence is just like giving the immune system a free lunch!

Carylic acid is also sometimes known as octanoic acid (because it is an 8-carbon substance) and is found in coconuts and breast milk.

Caprylic acid is an antimicrobial pesticide used as a food contact surface sanitizer in commercial food handling establishments on dairy equipment, food processing equipment, breweries, wineries, and beverage processing plants. It is also used as disinfectant in health care facilities, schools/colleges, animal care/veterinary facilities, industrial facilities, office buildings, recreational facilities, retail and wholesale establishments, livestock premises, restaurants, and hotels/motels. In addition to being an algaecide and bactericide, caprylic acid is a known fungicide.

Capsules (500 mgm) are readily available and not expensive.

Lufenuron

Here's An Even Newer Idea…

Lufenuron is a prescription-free, over-the-counter, totally harmless veterinarian remedy that kills Candida as effectively - but differently - than Diflucan (oral "azole" anti-fungal medicines), while putting no burden on liver and kidneys!

It makes holes in Candida's cell wall. It can cure vaginal yeast, oral Candida, Candida rashes and intestinal Candidiasis. More serious semi-systemic Candidiases such as IBS may need multiple treatments and are at least greatly improved.

A single treatment lasts one month. The Lufenuron is "loaded" into the fatty tissues over a period of five days, and then slowly releases, maintains tissue concentrations high enough to kill the Candida for one month. Anti-fungals such as Diflucan are harmful to the liver and kidneys. Lufenuron is not metabolized or eliminated by the liver or kidneys, but excreted through the feces.

Lufenuron is about as toxic as fruit juice. There are not side effects as such BUT: see the note on "die-off" which comes next.

Here's how it works: Lufenuron is an over-the-counter veterinary remedy available in pet shops under the name "Program". It is given to dogs or cats once a month, and it prevents flea larvae from growing into adult fleas by interfering with their Chitin synthesis. Chitin is the hard substance the exoskeleton of insects is made of.

What counts is that chitin is not just used by insects and arthropods, it also makes up about half of a fungus cell wall. And fungi - also Candida albicans - can't survive with half of their cell wall gone.

The effect it has on Chitin production (Chitin is not found in humans) makes this "off-label" use of Lufenuron an excellent broad-spectrum anti-fungal, successfully tested on a variety of animals in many countries around the world.

Lufenuron is not approved for use as an anti-fungal medicine in humans. This is not because of side effects, but simply because the manufacturer is not interested in getting this drug certified for use as an anti-fungal in humans. No human trials have therefore ever been initiated. However, Lufenuron has been used by countless thousands of humans, worldwide, and the results are impressive.

No reported side effects, and everyone with a verified Candida infection was either cured or improved strongly.

Download a free pdf book on Lufenuron and locate a supplier here: [http://lufenuroncandidacure.owndoc.com/lufenuron.pdf]

Big Surprise! Iodine

Not many people think of the antiseptic properties of iodine these days. It's still in the pharmacy, in a small bottle (1 oz.), to dab onto cuts and grazes.

However there is far more to iodine than this:

First, it's a natural immune booster and since we are all, according to official WHO figures, chronically deficient in iodine, it's good to take it.

You probably thought we have enough added to our salt and that was taken care of. Wrong!

The amount added to salt is pathetically low and not readily available biologically. Switching to iodized salt has seen average serum levels in the population plunge by more than half in recent decades. Why? Because doctors have spent those years telling patients not to eat salt!

But it's worse than that. Bromine and chlorine are lower molecular weight than iodine and so naturally displace the bigger (heavier) molecule. We add lots of chlorine to our water, so that's a problem. But we also now add bromine to bread.

In former times iodine was added to bread and worked well. Now manufacturers have not only stopped adding iodine to bread, they put in bromine instead. The bromine knocks out what little iodine is left in our diet and so the cycle worsens.

Trust me, you need iodine. You'll have to take care of this yourself.

But it gets better: iodine has strong anti-Candida properties. C. Orian Truss MD, whose name keeps recurring in this book, began using it in the 1950s.

He had read that potassium iodide solution could be used to treat Candida infestation of the blood. So he put the patient on six to eight drops of Lugol's solution four times a day and saw the patient promptly recover.

Soon afterwards Truss came across a female patient with a stuffy nose, a throbbing headache, vaginitis and severe depression; all her problems immediately cleared with iodine treatment. He saw a female patient who had been schizophrenic for six years with hundreds of electroshock treatments and massive drug dosages. By eradicating Candida, she soon recovered mentally and physically, and remained well.

In fact Truss saw a wide range of recoveries, including may psychiatric disorders, menstrual problems, hyperactivity, learning disabilities, autism, multiple sclerosis and auto-immune diseases such as Crohn's disease and lupus (LE).

In 1979 Truss produced a series of amazing and seminar papers in the journal of Orthomolecular Psychiatry, showing how Candida was a powerful cause of severe psychiatric disturbance.

- Orthomolecular Psychiatry, Volume 4, Number 1, 1978, pp. 17-37
- Orthomolecular Psychiatry, Volume 9, Number 4, 1980 pp. 287-301
- Orthomolecular Psychiatry, Volume 10, Number 4, 1981, pp. 228-238.
- Truss also wrote a useful book. It's still in print: "The Missing Diagnosis"

Lugol's Iodione Solution

Lugol's solution is named for the French physician J.G.A. Lugol. It was first introduced in 1829.

Lugol's iodine solution (5%) is often used as an antiseptic and disinfectant, for emergency disinfection of drinking water, and as a reagent for starch detection in routine laboratory and medical tests.

It consists of 5 parts of iodine crystals, 10 parts of potassium iodide and 85 parts distilled water (some formulas give 100 parts water, which is wrong). This is not the same as tincture of iodine. Tinctures contain alcohol and are much more concentrated.

Lugol's is sold in 100 ml bottles, also labeled Aqueous Iodine Oral Solution. Other names are iodine-potassium iodide and Markodine).

Test it first with one drop, to be sure there is no allergic reaction. If you are safe with iodine take 6 drops four times a day in liquid, such as fruit juice, or mixed with food.

Iodine is an oxidant and it is best to reduce the intake of antioxidants while using it; avoid vitamins A, C, E, grape seed extract or cysteine.

Continue for 3 weeks, but interrupt if you develop a serious reaction. Do not take the iodine for more than 3 weeks as that interferes with thyroid activity. If necessary repeat the course after several months.

You can buy Lugol's here, using PayPal or a CC: http://www.onlinegeneralstores.com/healthbeauty/iodine/iodine.htm

Or here (UK): http://www.healthleadsuk.com/supplements/liquid-concentrates-solutions-etc/lugols-iodine-30ml.html

or here (Australia): http://health.centreforce.com/health/lugols.html

Colloidal Silver

Colloidal Silver is one of the oldest remedies and can be traced as far back as the ancient Greek and Roman Empires. It is non-toxic, non-addictive and free of side effects.

It is thought to kill an average of 650 different organisms. This is staggering when compared to the 6 of a standard antibiotic!

It is safe for adults, children, animals and pregnant and nursing women. It can be applied topically and internally and has no reaction with other medications.

Typical maintenance use:

- 2-10 mls daily.
- Or one to four teaspoons (5mls).

In times of need, up to 25mls daily can be administered. In very serious health conditions, doses up to 500mls may be taken safely.

Some of the reported uses of colloidal silver are:

- Acne, Arthritis,
- Athlete's Foot,
- Bacterial infections,
- bladder infections
- Candida Albicans,
- Chronic Fatigue Syndrome
- Diabetes,
- diarrhea
- Eczema
- Intestinal disorders
- Prostate disorders
- Salmonella infection,
- septic ulcers, sunburn
- Yeast infections

Hydrogen Peroxide Therapy

Hydrogen peroxide (H_2O_2) is only one of the many components that help regulate the amount of oxygen getting to your cells. H_2O_2 is required for the production of thyroid hormone and sexual hormones.

It stimulates the production of interferon and dilates blood vessels in the heart and brain and it also improves glucose utilization in diabetics. The closer you look at hydrogen peroxide, the less surprising it becomes that it can help such a wide variety of conditions.

So, you may ask how H_2O_2 therapy will help Candida sufferers. The answer is very simple: H_2O_2 works against all anaerobic organisms which use carbon dioxide (CO_2) and these include all viruses, mutated Candida, gangrene and bacteria.

H_2O_2 is of little benefit when taken orally since it must enter the bloodstream directly. It is infused into the circulatory system intravenously for approximately ninety-minutes during which time the H_2O_2 spreads through the entire body reaching all cells.

On the cellular level it kills, or severely inhibits the growth of, anaerobic organisms (bacteria and viruses that use carbon dioxide for fuel and leave oxygen as a by-product).

Conditions that can be treated with H_2O_2 include all conditions that can be treated with antibiotics, but without the serious toxicity often associated with synthetic antibiotics.

Some of these conditions are Candida (yeast), viral infections, influenza, the common cold, sinus infection, Epstein-Barr virus and gangrene.

H_2O_2 therapy is a specialized therapy and should only be considered in cases where the Candida infection seems to persist over a prolonged period of time. As always, we recommend that you speak to your doctor or natural health practitioner before adding any supplements to your diet.

Taking Hydrogen Peroxide Safely

Be aware: hydrogen peroxide is potentially dangerous. As with so many things the toxicity is in the dose.

Use only food-grade hydrogen peroxide, to avoid toxic contaminants. But this is 35% strength and you MUST dilute it first, down to 3%, for safety reasons (one ounce food-grade to ten ounces of distilled water (1 in 11) = approximately 3%.

Never take hydrogen peroxide with food in your stomach. For most people this means an hour and a half either side of food. However if you feel a little nauseous after taking the H_2O_2 it could be because you haven't left it long enough.

Hydrogen peroxide is extremely active, chemically (that's why we take it) but that means it will interact with all kinds of foods and supplements, producing super-oxide free radicals. This can inflame the lining of your stomach. It also interacts with iron, copper, silver or manganese, so if you are supplementing these minerals, stop them a day before commencing H_2O_2 therapy.

Dosage Protocol

Use a 5-ounce (150ml) glass of distilled water as your carrier. Do not try to take a whole day's dose at once; split it: 3 times a day. As you increase the amount of drops increase the amount of water.

Day Number	Number Of Drops of 35% in a glass of water
1	3 drops, 3 times per day
2	4 drops, 3 times per day
3	5 drops, 3 times per day
4	6 drops, 3 times per day
5	7 drops, 3 times per day
6	8 drops, 3 times per day
7	9 drops, 3 times per day
8	10 drops, 3 times per day
9	12 drops, 3 times per day
10	14 drops, 3 times per day
11	16 drops, 3 times per day
12	18 drops, 3 times per day
13	20 drops, 3 times per day
14	22 drops, 3 times per day
15	24 drops, 3 times per day
16	25 drops, 3 times per day

For rampant Candida, start slowly, at 1 drop 3 times per day, then 2 drops 3 times per day. Then onto the above schedule.

Maintenance

After you have completed a 16 day protocol (maximum), you must reduce your intake to a maintenance dose. Do NOT try to continue beyond 16 days.

The frequency of Hydrogen Peroxide dosage should be reduced as follows;

- 25 drops once every other day, 4 times.
- 25 drops once every third day for 2 weeks.
- 25 drops once every fourth day for 3 weeks.

Taking vitamin E (either through foods or supplements) logically will help your body make better use of the extra available oxygen.

If you want to know more about so-called bio-oxidative therapies, read Medical Miracle by William Campbell Douglass MD.

Cathelicidins Research

A study was taken into anti-fungal activity of cathelicidins and their potential role in Candida albicans skin infection.

Cathelicidins have broad anti-microbial capacity and are important for host defense against skin infections by some bacterial and viral pathogens. This study investigated the activity of cathelicidins against Candida albicans.

The human cathelicidin LL-37, and mouse cathelicidin mCRAMP, killed C. albicans, but this fungicidal activity was dependent on culture conditions. Evaluation of the fungal membrane by fluorescent dye penetration after incubation with cathelicidins correlated membrane permeabilization and inhibition of fungal growth.

Anti-fungal assays carried out in an ionic environment that mimicked human sweat and with the processed forms of cathelicidin such as are present in sweat found that the cleavage of LL-37 to forms such as RK-31 conferred additional activity against C. albicans. C. albicans also induced an increase in the expression of cathelicidin in mouse skin, but this induction did not confer systemic or subcutaneous resistance as mCRAMP-deficient mice were not more susceptible to C. albicans in blood-killing assays or in an intradermal infection model. Therefore, cathelicidins appear active against C. albicans, but may be most effective as a superficial barrier to infection.

Mushrooms

Ironically, mushrooms (a kind of fungus) may have beneficial properties treating Candida though, as usual, the ignorant amateurs rant against anything in the fungus family (not really related, except distantly, to the yeasts).

Mushrooms, as you may know, produce lots of beta-glucans, which are recognized today as powerful immune stimulants. The turkey tail mushroom (Trametes versicolor) produces powerful Krestin and PSK, beta-glucans which have been used to destroy cancer.

The maitake mushroom (Grifola frondosa) contains compounds that specifically inhibit or destroy Candida albicans. It is thought that the several phytochemicals found in Grifola frondosa weaken the cell wall of the Candida albicans organism and make it more vulnerable to neutrophil attack.

As the "Candida vicious cycle" starts with poor immune function, an agent that stimulates impaired immune function could go a long way to break the chain. The objective of this study was to begin examining Grifola frondosa as such a potential cycle breaker.

In one five-month study, a strain of Grifola frondosa was examined for its ability to reduce symptoms in women with normal immune systems suffering persistent, chronic vaginal Candida infections.

It was a small study (22 women) sponsored by a British womens' magazine.

Twenty-two women were invited to take part in the study and were followed up at monthly intervals to monitor changes in their symptoms. Nine women withdrew from the study after the first month. Thirteen continued until the fifth month.

All respondents remaining in the study showed improvement in the severity of their symptoms. The range of improvement was between 7% and 80%. The results suggest that the strain of Grifola frondosa (Maitake) has a role in the control of chronic vaginal Candida albicans proliferation (Thrush) in normal women.

Another one to try is the Reishi mushroom (Ganoderma lucidum), also known to the Chinese as Lingzhi. It peroduces a protein compound called ganodermin which has measurable anti-Candida effects.

The fact that some mushrooms have a favorable impact on the condition refutes disinformation floating around the world of alternative medicine, that mushrooms are very bad for Candida patients!

It's a myth!

Essential Oils

Another important group of natural healers are the so-called "Essential Oils". This doesn't mean you have to have them; it means they are made from the odorous "essences" of the respective plants!

At the start of the 20th century, essential oils were the best antibiotics available to doctors and patients. Oregano was probably the star among these.

Oregano Oil (Origanum vulgare)

This oregano (also known as Greek or Mediterranean oregano) is not the culinary herb but a wild relative from the eastern Mediterranean.

When oregano oil was first tested in 1910 it was described as "the most powerful plant-derived antiseptic known" (H. Marindale). It has been found effective both in killing multiple bacteria, molds and yeasts and preventing their growth.

Oregano oil is the 'best of the best' active essential oils providing the amazing results in treating infectious diseases (P. Belaiche). It has been considered the closest to an ideal antibacterial agent.

Oregano oil has been tested against a variety of pathogenic microorganisms and is found to exert a high degree of anti-fungal, anti-parasitic, anti-viral and antibacterial actions. Oregano is such a potent anti fungal agent that it is capable of destroying even resistant fungal forms.

You can get oregano oil from almost anywhere. The active ingredient is carvacrol or isopropyl-o-cresol. Look for preparations with a high content (75% or more) of carvacrol. If the content is really high, oregano has been shown to be more effective than Nystatin against Candida (a leading drug for fungal infection that was explained in the previous).

Dose: 0.2 – 0.4 ml. twice daily, in an enteric coated form (otherwise you will get bad heartburn).

If you must use drops, dilute them with water or juice and build up slowly, starting with 1 drop 3 times a day.

Clove Oil (Syzygium aromaticum)

I found a great paper from 2006, showing great value in clove oil, carried out at the University of Porto, in Portugal.

The composition and antifungal activity of clove essential oil, obtained from Syzygium aromaticum, were studied. The clove oil analysed showed a high content of eugenol (85.3 %).

Tests were carried out to investigate the action of clove oil and eugenol against Candida, Aspergillus and other fungus strains.

According to the researchers, clove oil and eugenol caused a considerable reduction in the quantity of ergosterol, a specific fungal cell membrane component. They concluded that clove oil and eugenol have considerable antifungal activity against clinically relevant fungi, including fluconazole-resistant strains, deserving further investigation for clinical application in the treatment of fungal infections. [Pinto, E., Vale-Silva, L., Cavaleiro, C., Salgueiro, L. (2009). Antifungal activity of the clove essential oil from Syzygium aromaticum on Candida, Aspergillus and dermatophyte species. J Med Microbiol 58: 1454-1462]

Mountain Savory (Satureja Montana)

Mountain savory is great too. One important study examined in vitro antimicrobial activity of the essential oils of the aerial parts of Satureja montana L. and Satureja cuneifolia. The major compound of S. montana oil was the phenolic monoterpene carvacrol (45.7%).

The maximum activity of savory oil was observed against Escherichia coli, MRSA and against the yeast (Candida albicans). The essential oil of S. cuneifolia was also found to inhibit the growth of medically important pathogens such as S. aureus and E. coli. Fungicidal activity for both oils against C. albicans and S. cerevisiae (food yeast) was also observed.

Cassia (Cinnamon)

Cassia is actually a variety of essential oil preparations. The classic oil is made from true cinnamon, Cinnamomum zeylanicum, from Sri Lanka (former Ceylon).

But most oil preparations today use so-called Chinese cinnamon, a different species.

I found a very interesting paper testing the benefits vs. the safety of Cassia spectabilis. It was a powerful anti-fungal, with clear anti-Candida possibilities. What's more it tested out very safe indeed. [Fungicidal Effect and Oral Acute Toxicity of Cassia spectabilis Leaf Extract, S Sangetha, Z Zuraini, S Sasidharan and S Suryani, Nippon Ishinkin Gakkai Zasshi, Vol. 49 (2008)   No. 4   pp.299-304]

Another study tested a combination of a specie Cinnamomum cassia, alone or combined with amphotericin B, a drug widely used for most indications despite side-effects was investigated (see chapter 3).

Cassia allowed a dramatic 80% reduction in the dosage of Amphotericin B needed to kill Candida. This is a way of saying Cassia oil was 5 times more potent than Amphetericin.

Extracts of another specie, Cassia alata are traditionally used in Ivory Coast, West Africa to treat bacterial infections caused by Escherichia coli (E. coli), and fungal infections caused by Candida albicans and dermatophytes (athlete's foot, etc.)

An important study from the Department of Biology, at the Chinese University of Hong Kong, China looked at strais of Cinnamomum verum and Cinnamomum cassia.

An analysis of hydro-distilled Chinese cinnamon oil and pure cinnamaldehyde by gas chromatography/mass spectrometry revealed that cinnamaldehyde is the major component comprising 85% in the essential oil and the purity of cinnamaldehyde in use is high (more than 98%).

So this is different from carvacrol.

Both oil and pure cinnamaldehyde of Cinnamomum cassia were equally effective in inhibiting the growth of certain bacteria, but also fungi, including yeasts (four species of Candida, C. albicans, C. tropicalis, C. glabrata, and C. krusei), filamentous molds (4 isolates, three Aspergillus spp. and one Fusarium sp.) and dermatophytes (three isolates, Microsporum gypseum, Trichophyton rubrum and T. mentagraphytes).

I like this study!

Black Seed Oil

Black seed oil is not often included in Western reviews of essential oils. Maybe there is a certain amount of prejudice in this. But I think black seed oil could stand as high as Oregano oil and does not taste as repelling.

Black seed oil (Nigella sativa) has been known for centuries in Middle East countries. The black seed is known in Arabic as the habbutual barakah (the seed of blessing). It is sometimes called the Black Cumin Seed, however this is not the same as Black Cumin which the Indians refer to as Jeera/Zeera

The Prophet Mohammad stated in his "Hadith" that black seed oil cures every illness except death. A small phial of it was apparently found in the tomb of Tutankhamen.

Now modern science has come to its support. Researchers around the world have confirmed the anti-bacterial and anti-mycotic effects of black seed oil. Health practitioners in various countries around the world are using the oil against inflammation of all sorts as well as fungi infections.

Black Seed extracts have been found to stimulate bone marrow and immune cells, raise interferon production and increase B cells (which produce antibodies). Good against any infectious organism, in other words.

Black seed dose

A teaspoonful 3 times a day of the oil. It's bitter and irritating but can be mixed with tea, coffee, carrot juice, yoghurt or other carriers. For respiratory infections it can be rubbed in the chest; for sinusitis and catarrh, 3- 4 drops in each nostril.

General use

Ibn Senna known in the West as Avicenna (980-1037 AD) the Persian-born Islamic philosopher and physician who wrote the great medieval medical text, described the power of the black seed to stimulate the body's energy and banish fatigue.
A teaspoon of black seed oil mixed in a glass of orange juice with breakfast keeps you active all through the day. A teaspoon of black seed oil mixed in a hot drink after supper gives you a quiet sleep all through the night.

In one study, the anti-fungal activities of extracts of black seed were tested against eight species of dermatophytes, otherwise know as skin fungus.

The results revealed the potentiality of black seed as a source for anti-dermatophyte drugs and support its use in folk medicine for the treatment of fungal skin infections.

A further Turkish study, implemented at the Agricultural Faculty of the University of Erzurum in 1989, has also proved the antibacterial and anti-fungal qualities of black seed oil.

CHAPTER 5

Herbal Remedies

In this section, I have selected some excellent herbal and similar remedies that have shown to help Candida sufferers. Along with a food elimination diet (see the section on which foods to avoid) and the correct foods to eat (see section above on the best foods to eat), using these remedies to cleanse your body from a Candida overgrowth will certainly put you on a road to a speedy recovery.

Wormwood (Artemisia annua)

Recent research has found Wormwood to be extremely potent against the Candida Albicans fungal infection.

Gerald Green, a renowned medical herbalist, tried many well know anti-Candida remedies on his patients and found them all to be relatively ineffective compared with Wormwood.

Wormwood helps Candida sufferers by strengthening the immune system from the cell level up. This then helps people to overcome the primary cause of the Candida infestation fungal stage (a low and damaged immune system).

Wormwood capsules should be taken with water, three capsules twice a day for the first month, and three capsules daily for subsequent months.

Wormwood also:
- Invigorates and stimulates the whole digestive process.
- Helps with indigestion, when the cause is insufficient digestive juices.
- Anti-parasitic
- Anti-inflammatory

Wormwood treatment is one hundred per cent natural, which is great news for the patient. However a couple of days after starting treatment, most patients suffer from something called Herxheimers Syndrome (see above).

This only lasts 1-3 days, after which the patient suddenly feels a lot better, and will continue to improve quickly. Even though it is not pleasant, it is in effect a very good sign as it proves that the body is responding to treatment.

Olive Leaf Extract

Known as nature's protector, Olive leaf extract is:

- A natural, safe and effective alternative to antibiotics
- Highly beneficial for all types of infection
- A non-toxic way to strengthen immunity

US research at the Upjohn Company, published by the American Society for Microbiology, found that Olive leaf extract's active components, elenol acid and calcium elenolate, inhibited the growth of every virus, bacteria, fungi and protozoa they were tested against and this included the Candida fungus.

Research conducted at the Robert Lyons Clinic in Budapest, Hungary demonstrated such positive results against a range of infections that Olive Leaf Extract is now used by the Hungarian Government as an official anti-infectious disease remedy.

The study included over 500 patients suffering from a variety of conditions including tonsillitis, pharyngitis, pneumonia, bronchitis, pulpitis, leukoplakia, stomatitis, herpes, bacterial skin infections and Helicobacter pylori, all of which responded extremely well to treatment with Olive Leaf Extract.

As increasing number of positive results using Olive Leaf Extract are continuously reported. As such, excitement grows about its application in many infectious conditions and in people with compromised immune systems.

Research indicates Olive Leaf Extract could be useful in conditions such as:

- Chronic or recurrent viral or bacterial infections (e.g. colds, flu, sore throat, etc.)
- Candida, tinea, other yeast and fungal problems
- Parasitic infestation.
- Gut dysbiosis (leaky gut).
- Compromised immune systems

Olive leaf extract should be taken as such: 3 capsules daily (300mg).

This can then be increased to 3 capsules twice daily during times of extra need or when an acute infection occurs.

Lavender

Lavender is an herb rich in history and culture. Long prized for its healing properties, written records of the use of lavender for medicinal purposes date back as far as 60AD and the writings of Dioscorides.

In ancient Rome lavender was recognized for its healing and antiseptic qualities, its ability to deter insects, and for washing. In fact, its name stems from the Latin "lavare", meaning to wash.

In Medieval times lavender crosses were hung from doors to ward off evil and to safeguard against disease. In London, people wore bunches of lavender tied to their wrists to protect them from the Plague.

During the First World War, when modern antibiotics were sparse, lavender was used to dress wounds and helped to heal scar tissue and burns. Since then lavender has continued to be popular, and not only for medicinal purposes.

Lavender is renowned for its antibiotic properties. Studies have shown that the essential oil of lavender, particularly when combined with Geranium oil, is capable of killing some Staph infections.

Other studies have reported that lavender is good for treating ear infections, and is mild enough to treat such symptoms in children. Recently, four new chemicals have been isolated from lavender plants, and are believed to be beneficial for the treatment of Candida.

Grapefruit Seed Extract (liquid drops)

GSE is very effective for some people against Candida, although it would not be my first choice as an anti-fungal. Grapefruit seed extract should always be consumed in between every meal. If you feel any bloating, diarrhea, or constipation, try taking it in capsule or power form.

Here is how you should split the dosage of GSE:

- **Days 1-4:** Take 10 drops twice daily mixed with juice (veggie juice works best).
- **Days 5-10:** Take 15 drops twice. If you are taking capsules, take one 3 times a day.
- **Days 11-30:** Take 15 drops 3 times a day, or 2 capsules 3 times a day.

Gradually increase your dosage for a month, and then switch to a probiotic. 3-4 months with this regimen should reduce symptoms of candida dramatically

Aloe vera

Aloe gel is an oldie but universal goody. It has a place. You can apply it to external Candida infections, such as diaper rash or male genital yeast infections. Aloe vera gel is generally safe when applied topically and always feels soothing.

For intestinal Candida, which is what we are interested in, swallow 2- 3 ozs. (1/4 cup) of the juice daily.

For oral Thrush, which can be very unpleasant, rinse and gargle with Aloe. Be sure to spit out, to expel the infectious deposits rather than swallowing and passing them to the digestive tract.

White Tea Extract Research

On May 25, 2004 new studies conducted at Pace University indicated that White Tea Extract (WTE) may have prophylactic applications in retarding growth of bacteria that cause Staphylococcus infections, Streptococcus infections, pneumonia and dental caries.

This is what researchers stated when they presented their findings:

"Past studies have shown that green tea stimulates the immune system to fight disease," says Milton Schiffenbauer, Ph.D., a microbiologist and professor in the Department of Biology at Pace University's Dyson College of Arts & Sciences and primary author of the research. "Our research shows White Tea Extract can actually destroy in vitro the organisms that cause disease. Study after study with tea extract proves that it has many healing properties. This is not an old wives tale, it's a fact."

White tea was more effective than green tea at inactivating bacterial viruses. Results obtained with the bacterial virus, a model system; suggest that WTE may have an anti-viral effect on human pathogenic viruses. The addition of White Tea Extract to various toothpastes enhanced the anti-microbial effect of these oral agents.

Studies have also indicated that WTE has an anti-fungal effect on Penicillium chrysogenum and Saccharomyces cerevisiae. In the presence of WTE, Penicillium spores and Saccharomyces cerevisiae yeast cells were totally inactivated. It is suggested that WTE may have an anti-fungal effect on pathogenic fungi.

Several findings in the new study are of particular interest:

- The anti-viral and anti-bacterial effect of white tea (Stash and Templar brands) is greater than that of green tea.
- The anti-viral and anti-bacterial effect of several toothpastes including Aim, Aquafresh, Colgate, Crest and Orajel was enhanced by the addition of white tea extract.
- White tea extract exhibited an anti-fungal effect on both Penicillium chrysogenum and Saccharomyces cerevisiae.
- White tea extract may have application in the inactivation of pathogenic human microbes, i.e., bacteria, viruses, and fungi.

It has been surprising to researchers and doctors that white tea was shown to be more powerful than green tea.

Green tea is produced from the leaves of the evergreen plant Camellia sinensis. The major active ingredients of green tea are polyphenolic compounds, known as catechins.

Most famous of the is epigallocatechin gallate (EGCG), which makes up about 50% of the total amounts of catechins in green tea but there are several others that are powerful antivirals.

But white tea extract seems to be even more powerful, according to a 2004 study conducted at Pace University. Researchers found that White Tea Extract (WTE) may have prophylactic applications in retarding growth of bacteria, viruses and fungi. Their findings were presented at the 104th General Meeting of the American Society for Microbiology (listed above).

Moreover, the anti-viral and anti-bacterial effect of several toothpastes including Aim, Aquafresh, Colgate, Crest and Orajel was enhanced by the addition of white tea extract.

White tea was more effective than green tea at inactivating bacterial viruses. Results obtained with the bacterial virus, a model system; suggest that WTE may have an anti-viral effect on human pathogenic viruses.

While we are on with teas, let's look at Taheebo tea (Pau D'Arco) and Tea Tree Oil.

Other Stuff To Consider

Listen, there are LOTS of these alternative remedies. Here are some more to Google and give consideration to:

- Barberry (Berberis Vulgaris) Suma (Pfaffia Paniculata)
- Black Walnut Chaparral Echinacea/Golden Seal Combination Red Clover
- Propolis

All have been shown to have at least SOME anti-Candida effect.

Now A True Miracle...

Quinton Marine Plasma (QMP)

A surprising and little known way of transforming your terrain back to health.

So what is Quinton? Super sea water!

Not just any old sea water. It's special vortex water from certain algae blooms in the oceans, that are very rich in nutrients. It seems to have energetic properties too, above and beyond the mere presence of rare minerals etc.

The floor of our oceans is indescribably rich in minerals. Think about this: EVERYTHING that ever lived and died goes into the water system, down the rivers and ultimately finds its way to the ocean. Added to that is all the ocean life which lives, dies and is recycled, all the plankton, corals, fish, feces, EVERYTHING, which falls to the ocean floor as organic debris.

There is thick mud at the bottom of the ocean that contains dense nutrients and some minerals that are otherwise incredibly rare, like iridium, osmium, yttrium and so on. In fact pretty well the whole periodic table of substances is down there.

But it doesn't just stay on the ocean bed, lost to the biosystem. Quite the contrary. This nourishing mud is carried around the ocean floor by submarine currents which have only recently begun to be understood. There are certain places where this nutrient deposit wells up to the surface. Giant surges of ocean currents that we call convergences stir up the seas and bring the nutrients back to the surface bio system.

The polar oceans are classic sites for this. The huge bloom of algae that takes place in the Arctic and Antarctic every year yields a staggering abundance of life where the ocean, literally, changes color due to the density of life it carries.

This bloom is so rich it feeds the greatest animals of all: the whales. So much nutrition is absorbed into the biosystem at these sites in the summer time that whales can double their weight and deposit enough fat or blubber to live on it through the winter months.

The polar regions are not the only upsurges, however. In fact they can take place anywhere; typically along continental coastlines.

Enter Mr. Rene Quinton

Rene Quinton (pronounced cahn-ton) was a Frenchman, a doctor, biologist, biochemist and physiologist. At the end of the nineteenth century he discovered the healing merits of marine plankton plasma bloom, drawn from deep ocean water upsurges (about 10 metres depth).

It became a therapeutic sensation.

It is a little known fact that by 1907 Quinton had established 69 Marine Dispensaries and the product was already saving countless lives throughout the deadly pandemics of the early 20th century (tuberculosis, typhoid, cholera, syphilis, influenza).

Quinton's marine plasma (or QMP) was considered so effective for a wide range of common afflictions that is was reimbursed under two French laws, including Social Security. It was, of course, absurdly cheap.

When Quinton was finally buried in 1925, his fame had reached such proportions that tens of thousands of men, women and children, not to mention generals, dignitaries and statesmen, attended the funeral. Yet we have never heard of him. How can that be?

I think partly the rise of antibiotics starting in the 1930s is to blame. Doctors put more faith in the new drugs than older "simple" cures. Plus, in the latter half of the 20th century, Quinton marine plasma came under attack in France from the pharmaceutical industry.

However, Quinton manufacture did not fold up. The operation was moved to Spain and thanks to the more liberal scientific climate in Spain it has survived until today.

Now QMP has arrived in the US and is being sold by Original Quinton of Buena Park, CA.

Inner Terrain

The magic of QMP lies in the fact that it mimics our healthiest inner fluids, the so-called terrain: extra cellular, intracellular and interstitial fluids. In fact it is so good that animals can have their entire blood plasma volume replaced by QMP and they survive just fine. This is super-rich nutrient sea water bloom, not just the stuff you paddle in on the beach, OK?

You will readily see then that QMP is very safe, helps stabilize the internal milieu, provides every conceivable nutrient mineral and provides low concentration homeopathic-type mechanisms for healing. It's a miracle!

The "indications" (reasons to use it) are manifold and include: childhood gastroenteritis, poisoning, malnutrition and eczema; anemia, asthma, exhaustion, anti-aging, dysentery, tuberculosis and atherosclerosis; uterine and vaginal infections; rhinitis, sinusitis, respiratory allergies; skin allergies, dermal infections, histaminic reactions and psoriasis; energy restoration; bio-terrain restoration and burns.

I have even found that dentists can use it to save teeth, by injecting this healing balm into the surrounding gums. The abcesses and periodontal disease simply disappear.

There are DOZENS more uses.

The one that concerns YOU, reader, is that it is great for Candida/thrush. It can be swallowed, as a whole-body remedy or used as a vaginal douche! As such, it's great for correcting the poor terrain I've been talking about.

Whatever ever else you do about your Candida, be sure to include QMP as part of your regime.

How To Take It

QMP is taken by injections or orally. When injected, there is an isotonic form, which does not sting. Orally, the full-strength version is fine.

To take Quinton orally, snap off one end of the ampoule, put that end in your mouth, and as you suck, snap off the opposite end, so releasing the air pressure (a small plastic pad is provided, to be sure you don't cut yourself). Hold the liquid in your mouth for about a minute and then swallow.

Sprays work well for skin conditions.

It can even be taken by nebulizer, just breathed in. Or I find it very soothing for tired eyes. Just the whiff of "sea air" is very restorative to me!

It's so safe there are no real limits on the number of ampoules. It's only body fluid, after all! You can't OD on it like water (too much water will kill you).

QMP comes in 10 ml ampoules. 2, 3, 5, 10 ampoules are fine, depending on the seriousness of the complaint and if you are douching you will need the larger number to get enough in the pump. It's so cheap, cost is not an issue (less than $3 an ampoule)

Note that Quinton is not FDA approved for injection in the USA.

You can obtain it here: www.originalquinton.com

CHAPTER 6

Healthy Eating & Good Digestion

If I think I have yeast infection, what can I do?

This chapter is going to go into detail about diet and how to balance your body out. However, there are some simple things you can do right away.

If you are a healthy adult, you can try eating unsweetened yogurt or taking acidophilus. You can find this at your local health food store or drugstore. These treatments can help restore the balance between bacteria and fungus in your body and end the infection.

While I have oral thrush, what can I do to feel better?

- Cold liquids or frozen treats and juices may help to ease the pain of thrush
- Eat liquid foods that are easy to swallow
- Drink from a straw
- Rinse your mouth with a warm saltwater mixture (even better, use Quinton Marine Plasma, because that will help create an entirely healthier body, not just mouth cavity)
- For those territories where you can get ampoules of HEEL's "Traumeel" formula, I recommend that too.

Foods To Avoid

You should cut out all foods that contain yeast, or have been fermented or pickled, since these encourage the growth of Candida (see appendix for a fuller list of fermented foods).

Any Candida diet should strive to reduce or eliminate processed refined sugars and bleached flour. Eliminate meats treated with synthetic hormones or chemicals (eat organic).

Eliminate hydrogenated fats (peanut butter, baked goods and margarine, etc.). Reduce processed and refined foods as much as possible.

Specific foods to remove:
- Yeast extract
- Stock cubes
- Most bread
- Alcoholic drinks
- Cheese
- Black tea
- Cheese
- Bread
- Sugary fruits, such as banana, figs and dates. Avoid all dried fruits. Papaya, pineapple, grapefruit and all types of berries are fruits you should certainly eat.
- Pasta

- Sugar
- Chocolate
- And anything containing vinegar

As you can see, this removes a lot of the common foods that are usually eaten in our modern lifestyle.

My heart goes out to all of you suffering from this agonizing cycle of eating, bloating, discomfort, pain and cramps. And then it starts all over again. Or worse: It never goes away!

Starve The Candida Yeast

Remember is that you need to starve the Candida yeast. The best way to starve Candida is with a low carbohydrate diet. Carbs can be fermented, to provide energy for Candida and yeasts (alcohol is the result). A low carbohydrate diet produces a hostile environment in which Candida is unable to survive

Completely avoid all sweetened foods, honey, fruit juices, dried and fresh fruit. Also avoid milk and dairy products (except organic butter), because of their high content of the sugar lactose and antibiotic residues. You need this strict regime for at least a month but not permanently.

As a rule, eat plenty of salad, fish, poultry, meat and fresh vegetables (apart from the starchy ones like potatoes, parsnips and carrots). Try to obtain organic poultry and meat to avoid antibiotic residues.

When preparing meals, include liberal amounts of garlic, ginger and extra-virgin olive oil, and herbs such as rosemary, thyme, marjoram and lemon balm - which have strong anti-fungal properties.

Drink at least two liters of pure water every day, to help eliminate the toxins produced as the Candida dies off.

Replenish your beneficial bacteria by using a supplement of Acidophilus and Bifido-bacteria that guarantees at least 2 billion viable organisms per capsule. Take one capsule by mouth and, if not too painful, insert another capsule into the vagina every night before you go to sleep.

Start with your food elimination diet by incorporating the food groups in the section titled "the best foods to eat".

White Sugar

White sugar is one of the foods that Candida feeds off. It allows the infection to grow and spread like nothing else can. White sugar is a processed sugar. It is a sugar cane that has been stripped of all the original nutrients and essential fiber.

As such, white sugar contains no protein, no fat and no calcium. This means that is has no benefits at all to offer you body. It is one hundred percent chemical and actually harms your body when you consume it.

It does this because it stops the vitamins and minerals from your body. It also causes blood sugar levels to rise at an alarming rate.

Vegetetables

Some vegetables like raw garlic, onions, cabbage, broccoli, turnip and kale will actually directly inhibit the growth of Candida.

Buy your vegetables fresh and steam them. Add a little garlic for flavor (garlic is also helpful with Candida). Eat plenty of salads with raw salad vegetables such as celery and peppers to help detoxify and to help increase your energy.

Not only do vegetables starve the Candida of its sugar and mold diet, they also absorb fungal poisons and carry them out of your body.

Note: Keep starchy vegetables like potatoes and yams to a minimum.

Brussel Sprouts
Sprouts are known as a super food as they are highly nutritious, loaded with vitamins, easily digested and contain a lot of enzymes. They are great as internal cleansers in your body.

Using sprouts in your diet should be something you implement in order to bring your body back into balance and remove the yeast infection that you have.

If you have the inclination and the room to grow sprouts then you should consider doing so. There are a number of different types that can be grown. If you buy sprouts then ensure they are fresh, as they can become toxic when spoiled.

Non starchy vegetables
Non starchy vegetables are foods that you need to include in your new diet. These include things such as green peppers, celery, cucumber, lettuce, cauliflower, cabbage and spinach.

Non starchy vegetables are a great source of steady energy. This is because they release the energy into your body slowly and gradually (whereas refined carbohydrates give you a sudden influx).

[by starchy vegetables, I mean things like potato and yams).

Proteins

As part of your plan to starve the Candida yeast, feel free to eat plenty of high-protein meals. Foods like beef, chicken, fish and eggs are all good for you anyway and are almost completely free of sugars and mold. They will fill you up while restricting the Candid's appetite and growth. Other supplements can also help, whey protein being a good example.

Beans
Beans are a great source of clean protein. In order to get the best from beans you should soak them in water overnight once they are sprouted. They also need to be cooked for a long time

(and slowly) at a lower temperature. This cooking method will remove potential gases and help your body to easily digest the beans.

The type of protein that comes from beans can put stress on your digestive system unless you follow the instructions above.

Live yogurt cultures

Live yogurt cultures (or probiotics) are a class of supplement that helps your gut to repopulate itself with good bacteria. They are especially useful when suffering from Candida. The live bacteria in yogurt will crowd out the Candida yeast and restore balance to your system.

Good bacteria will also produce anti-fungal enzymes that can help you fight Candida.

Nuts and seeds

Another protein option that starves Candida and restricts its growth is seeds and nuts. Avoid peanuts, peanut butter, and pistachios as they tend to have higher mold content. Also consider soaking other nuts in water to remove any mold on the outside (spraying with a diluted grapefruit seed extract solution is even better).

Nuts such as almonds, pine nuts, pecans and Brazil nuts contain fatty acids that are good for the skin. They are also full of valuable nutrients and minerals. They are a good source of digestive protein.

Eat the nuts raw and in small quantities. Always store them in a cool place and eat them fresh.

Non-glutinous grains

Wheat and rye are best avoided for the first few weeks but there are other grains that you can eat. If you like toast in the morning, try millet bread instead of your usual brand. Rice can be eaten for a Candida diet, but get brown rice or preferably wild rice.

For cereal at breakfast, try a sugar-free variety with oat bran.

When bread is desired, you can always make soda bread (page 95).

Fruit

Previously, I have recommended that sugar-rich fruit needs to be eliminated from your diet. However, this does not mean all fruit should be eliminated. Your diet can still accommodate some papaya, pineapple, grapefruit and all types of berries. Strawberries, raspberries, boysenberries, etc. are all low in sugar.

The best diet and eating habits to form include nutrient-rich, organic, non- processed whole foods and plenty of fresh raw vegetables. You should also prepare most of your food yourself.

This diet is recommended as a guideline for someone who has never carried out an elimination diet before. Those with mild Candida symptoms may want to try it for 6- 8 weeks to evaluate if it helps. Those with severe symptoms should seek the help of a nutritionist or natural health practitioner with a case history of success with long term Candida sufferers.

Next, we are going to look at nutritional supplements that can help relieve the symptoms of Candida in addition to applying a food elimination diet.

Wheatgrass

Wheatgrass is probably the most powerful juice available to get anywhere. It contains huge amounts of chlorophyll which is the green pigment found in plants and is widely known for its great healing powers.

The reason to drink wheatgrass is because it cleans out the colon. It also alkalizes the blood, heals wounds, purges the liver, increases enzyme activity and also contains a lot of Vitamin E. It is also very rich in antioxidants.

You should take a serving of two ounces each day on an empty stomach. One other thing to pay attention to is not to drink too much too soon. If you drink too much then it can lead to hyper-detoxification, which will give you nausea.

More likely it would mean a wheat allergy!

Herb Teas

While fruit juices and water are some of the best things to drink, there are also other options that are open to you. Herb teas are made of freshly cut dried herbs. These have been known to have healthy and healing effects for thousands of years (For example, Chinese medicine has a recorded history of using green teas for many ailments and conditions).

Herbal teas are known for their medicinal values. The great thing about them is that they contain no caffeine and they are also highly therapeutic.

If you have problems with nausea or your appetite is suppressed, then some herbal teas can help you with this. Many herbal teas also supply you with minerals and vitamins. Others like comfrey are very nutritional.

If you are going to detoxify your body and follow the guidelines about diet, then you should drink a lot of herb tea in the process. This will supply your body with a great abundance of antioxidants and help it to regain balance.

In fact, there is almost no limit to the amount of herbal teas you can drink when detoxifying your body.

Some of the most therapeutic and nutritional herb teas are:

- Peppermint
- Parsley
- Comfrey
- Capsicum

- Chamomile
- Rose hips
- Kelp
- Cloves
- Alfalfa

If you are having problems with your digestion and want to increase your digestive system then use clove, cinnamon and nutmeg.

If you need to stimulate your bowels then you should use licorice or cascara sagrada.

Cleaning Fruits and Vegetables

Unless all your fruits and vegetables are organic, they are going to contain a high amount of bacteria, pesticides and parasites. This is because of the modern way that foods are produced, farmed and given an extended life. These days it is very hard to find truly organic foods.

There are however some vegetables that are easier to find organic than others. Organic carrots and other vegetables are now readily available in most supermarkets and stores.

As I said, it's very hard to get away from agricultural chemicals. There are even some present in so called "organic" vegetables. The good news is that you can clean the vegetables to remove some of the parasites and chemicals.

One of the best methods to clean vegetables is with four teaspoons of salt and lemon juice in a sink full of cold water.

From here you can then soak the vegetables with water and ensure they are completely rinsed through.

Another thing that you can do to kill most of the germs is to put them into boiling water. This will kill most of the germs but is not very suitable for more fragile vegetables.

Soda Bread (If You Must!)

Here is the process and recipe for making soda bread. You need to avoid yeast in bread. Bread without yeast is called unleavened. Soda bread (using baking soda to create carbon dioxide, which expands and fluffs up the bread) is quite a good substitute.

The Irish do it wonderfully! This traditional Irish soda bread is surprisingly quick and easy to prepare. For one 8-inch loaf you will need:

- tsp butter/dairy – free margarine/oil
- lb/455 g flour
- tsp bicarbonate of soda/baking soda
- tsp salt
- oz/115-225g buttermilk/goat's milk/soya milk (water if you are stuck)

Note that buttermilk is fermented and is not suitable for any anti-yeast or Candida diet. Use other suggestions for the liquid.

- Preheat the oven to hot (475oF/220oC/Gas Mark 7).
- Grease a large baking tray and set it aside.
- Sift the flour, soda and salt into a large mixing bowl.
- Gradually beat in the buttermilk or other liquid. The dough should be smooth but firm.

If necessary add more and shape it into a flat round loaf, approximately one and a half inches thick and eight inches in diameter.

Place it on the baking tray and make a deep cross on the top of the loaf with a sharp knife. Place the loaf in the oven and bake it for 30 to 35 minutes or until the top is golden brown. Remove it from the oven and allow it to cool. Best served slightly warm.

The Best Nutritional Supplements

You can help stop Candida with effective nutritional supplements.

If you are currently taking antibiotics, steroids, anti-ulcer medication or estrogen for other medical conditions, talk to your doctor about how you might safely reduce or stop these.

Start taking grapefruit seed extract (sold as 'Citricidal' by Higher Nature -- one capsule or ten drops in water, three times a day) to kill off the yeast. Alternatives are caprylic acid, which is derived from coconuts, or olive leaf extract.

Acidophilus
Replenish your beneficial bowel bacteria by taking a supplement of Acidophilus that guarantees at least 2 billion viable organisms per capsule (this should be kept in a refrigerator).

Aloe Vera Juice
Taking aloe vera juice, a tablespoon three times a day, will also help the good bacteria settle in and aid the healing of your gut lining - which can become damaged, irritated and 'leaky' as a result of Candida overgrowth.

Butyric Acid

Other supplements that aid this healing process are butyric acid (a fatty acid found in butter) and slippery elm (obtainable from herbalists as powdered bark). Take N-acetyl cysteine (500-1000 mg daily) which boosts your body's production of the amino acid glutathione and has powerful healing effects.

Butter Oil Protocol

This is very soothing for colonic Candida, especially if there is itching and staining around the anus, which are quite common and very irritating publicly. Butyric acid is found mainly in butter and butter oil. It can be administered rectally with good effect.

Insert a small amount rectally 3 times a week for a month (not enough to drip out again). Butter oil doesn't help much by mouth.

Often this will break the dysbiosis deadlock and probiotics can be discontinued as symptoms improve.

You can obtain pure butter oil from the Radiant Life Company: www.radiantlifecatalog.com

Milk thistle
Supplementing with milk thistle will help your liver break down these toxins, as will drinking plenty of water (drink at least two liters a day). You'll soon notice your symptoms disappearing and your 'brain fog' lifting - leaving you free to enjoy all that extra energy!

Boric Acid
Boric acid can often be very effective with severe infections. You can use two boric acid pills each day as pessaries. Just insert them gently into the vagina and let your body heat dissolve them.

Ensure that you don't have any allergies before using the pills. If the burning becomes severe then discontinue use.

Do NOT use chlorox to wash foods as some crazy nutritionists advocate. Organic foodstuffs plus chlorine create dangerous toxins called halogenated hydrocarbons, which are known to be carcinogenic and toxic. DDT and PCBs (polychlorinated biphenyls) are examples of halogenated organic compounds.

Tea Tree Oil

Tea tree oil is a very powerful anti-fungal agent and is completely natural. It is used for many conditions, such as helping with acne and other skin conditions (used in face wash). It is very effective at killing bacteria and is usually fine with any type of skin. Most people are not allergic to tea tree oil.

It can be used on almost any type of skin infection as well as those that penetrate the skin, such as yeast infection. It reduces the redness in the skin, eliminates puss and will also rejuvenate the skin.

What more, this treatment is antibacterial, antiviral and antiseptic. If you are going to use it, then buy the pure certified organic tee tree oil. [Clinical Microbiology Reviews, January 2006, p. 50-62, Vol. 19, No. 1]

Try it for ugly toenail infections too.

You can also try oil of bergamot (the nice smell in Earl Grey tea!). One study showed it was effective against dermatophytes, that is all skin and nail fungus. [Sanguinetti, M., Posteraro, B., Romano, L., Battaglia, F., Lopizzo, T., De Carolis, E., Fadda, G. (2007). In vitro activity of Citrus bergamia (bergamot) oil against clinical isolates of dermatophytes. J Antimicrob Chemother 59: 305-308]

But I recommend Pythium oligandrum (see page 53).

If you have sensitive skin then it is important that you do not use a 100% pure concentration of tea tree oil. The maximum concentration recommended is 20% tea tree oil diluted with jojoba oil.

A woman with a yeast infection should apply a few drops on a tampon before inserting it into the vagina. Be sure to dilute it first. A man can use a cotton bud and apply the tea tree oil to the infected area.

Summary

Fighting Candida is a battle you are going to win, mainly by banishing carbohydrates and sugary foods from your diet, eating fresh whole foods and by re-establishing healthy bowel flora with potent natural supplements.

Be prepared for some worsening of your symptoms, headaches or nausea, for a day or two - this is a good sign, as it means your body is successfully eliminating large quantities of dead yeast cells and their toxins from your body, and that you're on the road to recovery.

APPENDIX 1

The list below summarizes all the main yeast and fermentation products.

Fermentation and yeast Products

Substances that contain yeast, molds or ferments as basic ingredients :

- All Raised Doughs: Breads, buns, rolls, prepared frozen breads, sourdough and any leavened food.
- All Vinegars: apple, distilled, wine, grape, pear, etc. This includes all foods containing any vinegar, e.g. salad dressings, mayonnaise, pickles, sauerkraut, olives, most condiments, sauces such as barbecue, tomato, chili, green pepper and many others.
- All Fermented Beverages: Beer, lager, stout, wine, champagne, spirits. Sherries, liqueurs and brandies as well as all substances that contain alcohol, e.g. extracts, tinctures. Cough syrups and other medications, including homoeopathic remedies.
- All Cheeses" Including fermented dairy products, cottage cheese, natural, blended and pasteurized cheeses, buttermilk and sour cream.
- All Malted Products: Milk drinks that have been malted; cereals and sweets that have been malted.
- Ferments and Molds: Such as soy sauce, truffles and mushrooms.
- Antibiotics: Penicillin, ampicillin and many other '-illins" '-mycin' drugs and related compounds such as Erythromycin, Streptomycin and Chloramphenicol; tetracyclines and related derivatives; all the cephalosporin derivatives and all others derived from molds and mold cultures.
- Vitamins: B, B complex and multiple vitamins containing B complex. All products containing B6, B12, irradiated ergo sterol (Vitamin D). All health products containing brewer's yeast or derivatives.

Substances that contain yeast – or mold- derived substances:

- Flours that have been enriched (most)
- Milk enriched or fortified with vitamins
- Cereals fortified with added vitamins, i.e. thiamine, niacin, riboflavin, etc.

Substances that may contain molds as allowed contaminants commercially:

- Fruit Juices: canned or frozen. (In preparation the whole fruit is used, some of which may be moldy but not sufficiently so to be considered spoiled. Fresh, home squeezed should be yeast-free)
- Dried Fruits: Prunes, figs, dates, raisins, apricots, etc. Again, some batches may be mold-free but others will have commercially acceptable amounts of mold on the fruit while drying.

APPENDIX 2

TIPS FOR
AVOIDING
GE FOODS
(FROM WIKIHOW)

1. Become Familiar With The Most Common Applications Of Genetic Modification

These are the products (and their derivatives) that are most likely to be genetically modified:

- Soybeans - Gene taken from bacteria (Agrobacterium sp. strain CP4) and inserted into soybeans to make them more resistant to herbicides. See How to Live With a Soy Allergy for more information on avoiding soy products

- Corn - There are two main varieties of GE corn. One has a Gene from the soil bacterium Bacillus thuringiensis inserted to produce the Bt toxin, which poisons Lepidoteran (moths and butterflies) pests. There are also several events which are resistant to various herbicide. Present in high fructose corn syrup and glucose/fructose which is prevalent in a wide variety of foods in America.

- Rapeseed/Canola - Gene added/transferred to make crop more resistant to herbicide.

- Sugar beets - Gene added/transferred to make crop more resistant to Monsanto's Roundup herbicide.

- Rice - Genetically modified to resist herbicides; not currently available for human consumption, but trace amounts of one GM long-grained variety (LLRICE601) may have entered the food supply in the USA and Europe. More recently, golden rice, a different strain of rice has been engineered to produce significantly higher levels of beta carotene, which the body uses to produce vitamin A. Golden rice is still undergoing testing to determine if it is safe for human consumption. [http://news.bbc.co.uk/1/hi/sci/tech/4386933.stm accessed 3.45 pm BST 2/10/2010]

- Cotton - engineered to produce Bt toxin. The seeds are pressed into cottonseed oil, which is a common ingredient in vegetable oil and margarine.

- Dairy - Cows injected with GE hormone rBGH/rBST; possibly fed GM grains and hay.

- Aspartame/AminoSweet - Addictive and dangerous artificial sweetener commonly found in chewing gum and "diet" beverages. A building block of aspartame, the amino acid phenylalanine, is usually manufactured with the aid of genetically modified E. coli bacteria. This process has been used industrially in the USA for many years.

- Papayas

- Farm Raised Salmon

2. Buy Only Food Labeled 100% Organic

The US and Canadian governments do not allow manufacturers to label something 100% organic if that food has been genetically modified or been fed genetically modified feed. However, you may find that organic food is more expensive and different in appearance from conventional products. Also, just because something says "organic" on it does not mean that it does not contain GMs. In fact, it can still contain up to 30% GMs, so be sure the labels say 100% organic.

This applies to eggs, as well. Eggs labeled "free-range", "natural", or "cage-free" are not ecessarily GE-free; look for eggs to be 100% organic.
[http://truefoodnow.files.wordpress.com/2011/02/cfs-shoppers-guide.pdf accessed 3.45 pm BST 2/10/2010]

3. Recognize Fruit And Vegetable Label Numbers

If it is a 4-digit number, the food is conventionally produced.

If it is a 5-digit number beginning with an 8, it is GM. However, do not trust that GE foods will have a PLU identifying it as such, because PLU labeling is optional. [http://www.undoge.org/?p=25 accessed 3.45 pm BST 2/10/2010]

If it is a 5-digit number beginning with a 9, it is organic.
[http://missourifamilies.org/features/nutritionarticles/nut76.htm accessed 3.45 pm BST 2/10/2010]

4. Purchase Beef That Is 100% Grass-Fed

Most cattle in the U.S. are grass-fed, but spend the last portion of their lives in feedlots where they may be given GM corn, the purpose of which is to increase intramuscular fat and marbling. If you're looking to stay away from GMOs, make sure the cattle were 100% grass-fed or pasture-fed (sometimes referred to as grass-finished or pasture-finished). The same applies to meat from other herbivores such as sheep. There is also the slight possibility that the animals were fed GM alfalfa, although this is less likely if you buy meat locally. With non-ruminants like pigs and poultry that cannot be 100% grass-fed, it's better to look for meat that is 100% organic.

5. Seek Products That Are Specifically Labeled As Non-GM Or GMO-Free

However, it is rare to find products labeled as such. You can also research websites that list companies and foods that do not use genetically modified foods, but be aware that information is often incomplete and conflicting interests may not be declared.

6. Shop Locally

Although more than half of all GM foods are produced in the US,[8] most of it comes from large, industrial farms. By shopping at farmers' markets, signing up for a subscription from a local Community Supported Agriculture (CSA) farm, or patronizing a local co-op, you may be able to avoid GM products and possibly save money at the same time.

More and more small farms are offering grains and meat directly to customers, in addition to the usual fare (vegetables, fruit, herbs).

Inspecting non-GMO cabbage Shopping locally may also give you the opportunity to speak to the farmer and find out how he or she feels about GMOs and whether or not they use them in their own operation.

7. Buy Whole Foods

Favor foods that you can cook and prepare yourself, rather than foods that are processed or prepared (e.g. anything that comes in a box or a bag, including fast food). What you lose in convenience, you may recover in money saved and satisfaction gained, as well as increased peace of mind. Try cooking a meal from scratch once or twice a week--you may enjoy it and decide to do it more often.

8. Grow Your Own Food

This way you know exactly what was grown, and what went into growing it.

Made in the USA
Middletown, DE
12 October 2020

21709057R00057